Psychiatry for Primary Health Care in Uganda

Editor
Emilio Ovuga

MAKERERE UNIVERSITY
Kampala

FOUNTAIN PUBLISHERS
Kampala

Fountain Publishers
P.O. Box 488
Kampala
E-mail:fountain@starcom.co.ug
Website:www.fountainpublishers.co.ug

Makerere University
P.O. Box 7062
Kampala, Uganda

Distributed in Europe, North America and Australia by African Books Collective Ltd (ABC), Unit 13, Kings Meadow, Ferry Hinksey Road, Oxford OX2 0DP, United Kingdom.
Tel: 44(0) 1865-726686, Fax:44(0)1865-793298.
E-mail: abc@africanbookscollective.com
Website: www.africanbookscollective.com

First published 2006

ISBN 13: 978-9970-02-611-1
ISBN 10: 9970-02-611-9

Contents

Acronyms

AGOU	Association of Gynaecologists and Obstetricians of Uganda
AIDS	Acquired Immune Deficiency Syndrome
APRO	African Psycare Research Organisation
ASD	Acute Stress Disorder
CSF	Cerebro-Spinal Fluid
CCR	Criteria for Criminal Responsibility
CT	Computerised Tomography
EEG	Electro-Encephalography
ESR	Erythrocyte Sedimentation Rate
Hb	Heamoglobin
HIV	Human Immune Deficiency Virus
HMIS	Health Management Information Systems
IDP	Internally Displaced Persons
I.M.I.	Intra-Muscular Injection
MCHC	Mean Corpuscular Haemoglobin Concentration
MCV	Mean Corpuscular Volume
MRI	Magnetic Resonance Imaging
PCV	Packed Cell Volume
PTSD	Post-traumatic Stress Disorder
RBC	Red Blood Count
T3	Tri-iodothyronine
T4	Thyroxine
TPHA	Treponema Pallidum Hem-Agglutination
TSH	Thyroid Stimulating Hormone
VDRL	Venereal Diseases Research Laboratory
WBC	White Blood Count

Contributors

Abbo, Catherine, MB ChB, M. Med. (Psych.), works at the Forensic Psychiatry Unit, Butabika Hospital and Department of Psychiatry, Makerere University. Dr Abbo has conducted research in traditional medicine for which she has won an award for young researchers in psychiatry from the American Psychiatric Association. She has special interest in promoting collaboration with traditional healers in Uganda.

Birabwa, Harriet, MB ChB, M. Med. (Psych.), is a psychiatrist at Butabika Hospital and has special interest in affective disorders.

Maling, Samuel, MB ChB, M. Med. (Psych.), is the Head of Department, Psychiatry, Mbarara University of Science and Technology.

Nakasi, Grace, MB ChB, M. Med. (Psych.), is Senior Lecturer, Department of Psychiatry, Makerere University. She is the first child psychiatrist in Uganda.

Nakku, Juliet, MB ChB, M. Med. (Psych.), is a Psychiatrist at Butabika Hospital and has special interest in promoting women's mental health.

Ovuga, Emilio, MB ChB, M. Med. (Psych.), PhD, is Associate Professor of Psychiatry, Department of Psychiatry, Makerere University. He has a wide range of clinical and research interests, including neurology, suicidology, psychotherapy, community psychiatry and primary health care and conflict mitigation. Dr Ovuga is currently involved in developing a model of community mental health care delivery system for districts involving communities incorporated within existing district health care systems.

Wakida, John, RMN/RGN, Dip (Health Education), Dip (Nursing Administration), BA (SS) is Principal Nursing Officer at Butabika Hospital and is specialised in public administration.

Foreword

Untreated mental illness does impair the social and economic lives of affected individuals significantly. In the eyes of the public in Uganda, any individual who suffers from mental illness is not expected to regain his/her normal senses and return to normalcy. Contrary to this widely held belief, however, I have had the opportunity to witness people adequately recover from severe disorganising mental illness and regain good productive lives. There is no doubt in my mind that the course of severe mental illness can indeed be reversed for the better.

As rapid strides are being taken to develop mental health services in Uganda, the commitment of the mental health professional to heal the sick mind must be based on scientific evidence. To achieve this, the psychiatrist must, I believe, have a wide theoretical knowledge base and keep abreast with developments in the speciality of psychiatry, general medicine, and the politics and sociology of good clinical practice. Likewise general medical workers should make every effort to inform themselves about mental health issues in Uganda. I firmly believe that the optimal care of the mentally sick is certainly within the capability of every health care provider practicing in Uganda. This book has been written to enable the non-expert in the field of mental health to provide appropriate and optimal mental health care to those who suffer from mental illness in primary care where there may be no mental health specialist such as the psychiatric nurse or the psychiatric clinical officer.

To achieve this, the establishment of professional working relationships with health service users and their families is needed. Though patients come to the health care provider to receive care, they usually do so expecting that they will, in some way, participate in the process of receiving that care. This expectation is not unreasonable considering that the patient and his/her care-givers will be expected to comply with a range of medical instructions and expectations.

It is now standard practice to empower patients and or their care-givers in planning treatment protocols. Empowering patients and their families is expected to promote compliance among patients and their care-givers, reduce disability, improve economic productivity, and improve the quality of life of the patients.

This book has been written to foster quality health care and good quality of life for the mentally sick in Uganda. Guidelines covering a wide range of management issues have been presented. A first glance at the book might show that it has been prepared primarily for psychiatrists. I am aware, however, that the Government of Uganda has now fully integrated mental health in the national minimum health care package at all health units. This means that every health care provider working at any health unit will come in contact with at least one mentally sick patient at least once in a month. This book has been prepared to meet the needs not only of the mental health care provider but also those of the general health care provider in Uganda. It is my firm belief that the use of this book that addresses common mental health problems in primary health care will enable the primary heath care provider to provide clinical care to those suffering from mental disorder. I recommend the book as a quick reference book for every health care provider. The book should definitely be stocked on the shelf of every major health unit and health training institution in Uganda.

Professor Nelson K. Sewankambo
Dean, Faculty of Medicine
Makerere University

Introduction

EMILIO OVUGA

Between 15-40% of the general population experience some form of psychiatric disorder at any one time and 20-30% of primary care attendees do so primarily for emotional problems. Approximately 10-15% of psychiatric disorders presenting for treatment at health units in Uganda are due to physical disorder and 20% of patients with psychiatric illness have at least one general health problem requiring appropriate attention. Though mental illness is responsible for only 0.4% of total mortality, it causes considerable amount of disease burden and disability. Mental disorders, particularly depression, schizophrenia, alcohol and substance use disorders, and obsessive-compulsive disorders, all of which are common in Uganda, are among the leading causes of disease burden. Unfortunately the provision of mental health care is hampered by many factors including cultural concepts of aetiology and treatment, myths about mental illness, stigma, discrimination, denial, and acute shortage of mental health professionals.

The mentally ill are among the most vulnerable to abuse and the least respected members of the Ugandan society due to the nature of their condition. Mental illness affects the interests of both the patient and their respective families. However since the discovery of penicillin and chlorpromazine for the treatment of general paralysis of the insane and schizophrenia respectively, individuals who would otherwise be left to the mercy of nature can now lead normal and productive lives in society if appropriate and timely treatment is provided to the persons concerned. The care of the mentally ill should not the responsibility of mental health professionals alone but also that of the patients themselves, their families, the community, other health professionals and community agencies concerned with the welfare of those considered to be in need of social and health services. Psychiatric care thus requires teamwork and appropriate networking involving patients, their families, health professionals and community agencies. Appropriate and early psychiatric care improves the quality of life of the mentally sick. The guidelines contained in this book aim to: a) aid the process of providing appropriate care to those who are mentally ill b) protect the rights of patients c) facilitate the involvement of patients and their carers in the development of mental health care and d) protect mental health workers in the process of providing care.

Mental illness:

- Is very painful to the people affected and their families and requires correct treatment early to prevent further suffering.
- Can affect anyone, any time and any where.
- Can be controlled, treated and in some cases, cured.
- Is not due to witchcraft or wrongdoing on the part of the affected people or members of their clan.
- Can start suddenly over a short period of time or gradually over the course of a few months to one or two years.
- May lead to obvious changes in behaviour, self-care and habits, or may not result in any obvious changes at all until relatively late.
- May present disguised in the form of prevailing social, political or economic circumstances of the time.
- Must be accorded the same status in the health care delivery system as physical health.

The most important sign of mental illness is *change in behaviour pattern* in private or social life. The people most suited to recognise this are the family, friends or other close acquaintances who know the individual well.

This book is intended to help the primary health care provider learn about mental illness and provide appropriate care to the people affected by the condition. It is important to note the following points about mental health problems from the very start as one begins to learn about mental illness, its management, its prevention and the promotion of overall psychosocial wellbeing. Mental illness is the same as any other human health problem and deserves to be accorded the same attention from everyone as any other branch of clinical medicine.

The guidelines in this book have been developed bearing in mind the special socio-economic situation in Uganda. For instance although more effective drugs with fewer side effects are available in Europe and North America, these have not been included in the book because of their costs relative to the purchasing power of the Uganda shilling.

The guidelines recognise the often confusing and difficult relationship between the rights of the patient and those of his/her family and community. The health worker, and particularly the psychiatrist, must constantly evaluate the relative weight of the patient's rights against the rights of others around the patient. Individuals who suffer from the severe forms of mental illness (psychosis) suffer from loss of insight into their general as well as mental health state. Such persons will not have the capacity to seek treatment and will lack the ability to appreciate the harmful effects of their illness behaviour on others around them. Under such circumstances treatment and care will normally be provided under the provisions of the Mental Treatment Act, the Penal Code or the Magistrates' Courts Act. It is recommended that these guidelines should be used alongside the appropriate legal instruments.

Research in Uganda has shown that traditional (alternative) medicine as this assumes a central role in the provision of mental health services to the mentally sick. Accordingly a chapter has been devoted to this sector of the healthcare system in Uganda for the purpose of stimulating further research on traditional medicine and promoting collaboration between modern and traditional forms of healthcare.

It is hoped that this book will help in the process of advocacy and lobbying for mental health and its problems in Uganda, the promotion of patient compliance, prevention or reduction in the rates of illness relapse, and the protection of the dignity of patients and their carers.

SECTION I

General Principles in Mental Health Care Provision

1
Admission, Discharge and Referral of Patients

EMILIO OVUGA

Introduction

The majority of individuals with active symptoms of mental illness should receive treatment on outpatient basis. In a minority of cases admission for inpatient care is necessary for a rapid control of an acute psychiatric disturbance, permit observation of the clinical state to be made, allow for specialised laboratory investigations to be carried out, and to enable the family to rest from the impact of continuing psychiatric illness.

Admission

The following often necessitates admission to hospital for in-patient care:

- Violent, noisy, excited and irrational behaviour.
- Lack of care and protection for the patient.
- Self-destructive behaviour (risk of suicide).
- Need for in-patient supervision of medication.
- Need for in-patient observation and investigations.
- To make psychiatric observation of individuals who are suspected to have committed a crime.

Admission may be voluntary when the patient requests to be admitted to hospital or compulsory when the patient lacks insight into his/her mental state yet requires medical treatment or needs to be removed temporarily from the family for the protection of family members.

1. Record the reasons for admission after careful history taking.
2. Have the relevant admission forms filled and signed.

Referring psychiatric patient/client

Psychiatric disorders often complicate general medical disorders and up to 60% of general hospital patients who require some form of mental health service occupy beds. Conversely, at least 15% of psychiatric disorders are caused by an organic condition such as thyroid disease, infective process, nutritional deficiency, neurological disorder, etc.

Psychiatry deals with human problems including problems in interpersonal relationships. Individual psychiatric practice should therefore embrace a holistic principle in the provision of care not only aimed at the cure of illness episodes but also aiming at the promotion of good health, the promotion of compliance, prevention of future illness episodes and the reduction of the harmful effects of psychosocial stressors.

Indications for Referral

- Lack of facilities for investigations or appropriate clinical care.
- Lack of personal skills, experience or knowledge needed to provide care for a particular clinical condition.
- Suspected or diagnosed medical condition responsible for or in co-existence with the psychiatric illness.
- Suspected or diagnosed neuro-surgical disorder.
- Coma or injury the patient sustained following a suicide attempt.
- The patient is in need of other services such as legal aid, spiritual service, specialised psychotherapy, occupational therapy, rehabilitation, social casework and physiotherapy.

When Referring

1. Follow the guidelines concerning the protection of confidential information about patients.
2. Discuss with the patient, and or carer, the need for referral. Indicate in your clinical notes that such a discussion did take place.
3. Inform the patient and or carer of the likely outcome of the referral.
4. If you are only a member of a team providing care for the patient, the decision to refer should be taken by the team unless the referral is done as a life-saving emergency. Even then team members should be informed at the earliest opportunity thereafter.

5. Referrals from lower level health units to higher levels within the district should be signed by the respective officers in charge; all referrals to centres outside the district (to Regional or National Referral Hospital) should be signed by the Medical Superintendent or his/her appointed deputy.
6. Provide concise clinical information, which should include: history, clinical findings, and laboratory results, treatment so far provided by you or your team, and the reasons for referral.
7. Request for feedback information.
8. Indicate willingness to receive the patient back as necessary.
9. Refer according to protocols that govern patient referrals at your health unit. If no such protocols exist it is important that the health unit develops them in accordance with the code of current practice provided by the Ministry of Health.

When Receiving a Patient

1. Inform other team members of any new patients you have received.
2. Discuss with the patient and or carer the need for feedback to the referring doctor on clinical findings, treatment, and what the referring doctor or agency should do if they receive the patient back for follow-up.

Discharge

The patient may be discharged from hospital when clinical recovery is considered to have been effected on medication and other forms of therapy employed. Under existing legislation, a person who has been admitted to mental hospital can only be discharged after 365 days unless the Hospital Superintendent advises that the individual can be discharged before the legal period has elapsed. On other occasions, however, the patient or family may request discharge even before adequate clinical improvement. This is perfectly in order particularly if the patient was admitted informally, and not on any temporary legal order signed by the police or the magistrate. Moreover psychiatric care in primary care is unlikely to be offered in a gazetted mental hospital at the district level. If, however, the family of a patient who has been admitted under a legal order for admission in a gazetted hospital demands discharge, such request may be granted as a discharge against medical advice, and this should be indicated in the client's case file. In many cases, it is feasible to convince relatives and patients either in favor of more days in hospital or the use of out-patient review facilities till full recovery is achieved.

When can the patient be discharged?

This should be based on the outcome of regular clinical reviews which indicate a combination of the following clinical indicators depending on diagnosis:

- Disorganised behaviour has been brought under effective control
- Hallucinations have resolved
- Delusions have disappeared or are minimal
- Symptoms of depression are gone
- Suicidal risk has gone and the individual has no suicidal wish
- Underlying physical condition is cured
- Social relationships have been restored and the person interacts with the social environment normally
- The person has regained normal general habits
- Self-care has improved
- Sleep and appetite for food are normal
- The person participates normally in social and domestic work, functions and activities
- The individual has regained full insight into his/her mental health needs
- Intellectual functioning is back to normal or near normal

Caution

Some patients with manic illness, paranoid disorder or alcohol dependence problems can effective mask signs and symptoms of mental ill-health. When this happens and the individual relapses within 4 to 8 weeks as can be expected, you will need to be more careful in your future plans to discharge the persons concerned.

Steps to take in discharging patients

It is likely that at a district health facility the hospitalised patient may be nursed with the assistance of key family members. If this is the case the decision to discharge will be made jointly with the family members concerned and the patient based on the observations made by the family. Before you discharge the patient, take the opportunity to teach the patient and family members about early warning symptoms and signs such as lack of sleep, loss of appetite, restlessness, and the reappearance of specific symptoms associated with the mental disorder, etc.

Discuss in simple terms the course and likely outcomes of the condition on treatment as well as when the patient stops medication. Provide information on drug side-effects and how these can be controlled or prevented. Encourage normal activity and participation in usual domestic and social activities for the patient so as to prevent stigmatization, discrimination and social rejection.

If the patient's home is far from the hospital or the family lacks the means to be at the health unit during the course of hospitalisation, make a home visit to understand the situation at the patient's home. During the home visit take off time to provide information on the mental health problem, its treatment, course and outcome, treatment benefits and side-effects and what can be expected from the individual after he/she returns home. Secure the understanding, participation and contributions of the family in the promotion of the mental health of the individual outside hospital.

If the health facility has established a network of community volunteers in mental health, the family should be introduced to these to enhance the ability of the family to supervise medication and assure its access to drugs. Ensure that you provide clear instructions for follow-up and drug use. Be certain, however, that you do not delegate the clinical responsibilities of the health facility to the community volunteers.

2
Communication in Provision of Health Care

Emilio Ovuga

Communicating health information

The average patient wants to know about his/her condition, about what is going on, what is being done about it, what the results of investigations mean, what the chances are for cure, and what he/she should do to maintain good health. Lack of communication by the doctor is one of the commonest reasons for the loss of trust in the doctor and for poor compliance.

Communication Hindrance

Communication of useful health information may not be possible if:

(i) The patient has an acute and severe mental illness (psychosis) or has clouding of consciousness. It is advisable to hold information until the patient is in a position to comprehend it.

(ii) The patient lacks supporting social network and he/she is unable to benefit from the communication of information.

(iii) The nature of the health problem concerned is sensitive; the risk of open communication of the information far outweighs the benefits of withholding the information.

(iv) The patient does not wish to know about his or her condition.

Benefits of Information

Appropriate communication of health information should primarily be made to the patient unless the patient is a minor or is unable to receive and comprehend health information on account of impaired cognition, hallucinations or delusions. If the communication of health information is considered vital, such as the need to prevent an impending suicide attempt or risk of injury to other people, carers may be informed. The following are the benefits of communicating health information to patients and or their carers.

(i) The patient and or carer will develop a sense of being respected and cared for by the doctor.

(ii) The communication will serve as a means of empowering the patient and or carer to cope with illness, live with the illness, and help the patient or carer to avoid deterioration in the status of the health condition.

(iii) The patient and or carer will make informed decision and give informed consent to all medical procedures including investigations, formulation treatment plans, and referral to other health specialists.

(iv) The patient or carer will not feel that decisions have been imposed on them; the patient and or carer will own any decision made.

(v) Promotion of patient compliance.

(vi) Patient and or carer will understand the basis of medical advice.

(vii) Creation of awareness of the side-effects of medical procedures.

(viii) Creation of patient and or carer's co-operation.

Indications

Communication of health information is warranted under the following circumstances.

- Communication of chronic, debilitating or fatal illness, e.g. epilepsy, cancer HIV/AIDS, or mental illness
- Communicating opinion on a sensitive social or health issue, e.g. conjugal jealousy, HIV/AIDS status
- As a prelude to making a request, e.g. the need to make a report, or to provide health education, e.g. the aetiology, management and prevention of paranoid psychosis due to hypertension, alcohol abuse or typhoid fever.

Note that the list provided is not exhaustive.

Guidelines to the Communication Process

Do not underestimate the level of understanding of rural patients, and lack of education should not discourage you from passing vital health information to all patients who have no active psychosis or significant impairment of cognition. The belief and values systems of the patient might vary from yours but this fact should not deter you from communicating vital health information to the patient as part of your effort to provide the best care for your patients.

1. A number of leading questions may be put to the patient at the begining"*What did Doctor (so and so) say you suffer from? .... What about you? .... What do they call the condition you suffer from? What have friends said about your condition or illness? ... What do you think you suffer from?"*

   The patient and or carer will usually calmly receive the information when the communication is based on the patient's history. Note, however, that there are always two ways in which the patient and or carer might respond to the communication of health information. Patients may receive information with mixed feelings; denial; worry and fear; with emotional numbness; sense of relief; anger and frustration; and shock and sense of desperation. The following quotation from a carer illustrates the reaction of patients and carers: "The doctor said: basing on the symptoms available, it is AIDS. I felt like the doctor shot a bullet through my heart or my brother's (patient) heart." Care must therefore be exercised in selecting the most effective way of communicating sensitive health information. A balance must always be drawn between providing information for the good of the patient and not doing so.

2. Communication may be made in the following way as judged appropriate: *It is possible that I may be wrong. However based on the information available (you should list the salient features of the information), it appears to me that.....*

3. Pause and watch the patient silently for his/her response. Do not say anything until you get the cue to speak again.

4. Let the patient or carer express his/her emotions if this happens spontaneously at some stage, e.g. sign of shock, despair, fear, relief,

etc. Do not stop the patient or carer weeping if this happens for it will usually last no more than 2 minutes at most; weeping is healthy and it facilitates the relief of emotional tension.

5. Next provide reassuring information appropriate to the issue being discussed including treatment, the likely duration of treatment, the course of the illness, and the prognosis of the condition.

6. Any further information to be communicated will depend on the mood and response of the patient and or carer.

- Remember that the patient and or carer may be inattentive to much of what you might say, particularly after receiving illness information. You should therefore be tolerant and repeat yourself as often as necessary. Speak slowly and in simple language. Even then, do not be surprised if the patient forgets much of what you say.
- When the patient and or carer is ready, discuss possible strategies for coping.
- Give opportunity for the patient and or carer to ask questions; this will help you to remember any other information that you might have forgotten to provide.

When a patient and or carer declines to receive information, accept this as a natural human response and as the exercise of their right. Such refusal should not preclude the patient and or carer from receiving further care from you. Rather you should leave the door open for the patient and carer to contact you for additional care if they so wish. Indeed it is likely that the patient and or carer will seek the information from you at a later date when they are ready.

3

Professional Ethics in the Provision of Mental Health Services

EMILIO OVUGA

Rights of the mentally sick person

The mentally sick persons are human as anyone else. However owing to the nature of their illness, the mentally ill do not often get the quality health and social care they so badly need. Those who suffer from severe mental illness may lack the ability to take part in rational considerations in their interest, fail to give consent either way, and decisions may be made for them even though some of the decisions may be detrimental to their welfare. Despite this it should the duty or the health care provider to advocate safe, fair and equal treatment of the mentally ill, within the provisions of the constitution and mental health law for the purpose of promoting health, relief of suffering and the promotion of life for patients and family. In 1991, the United Nations General Assembly passed a resolution affirming for the rights of persons suffering from mental illness (United Nations, 1991).

The following rights of the mentally ill individual are derived from the Declaration of Madrid of 1996 and the United Nations resolution to underline appropriate mental health practice.

Psychiatric patients have a universal right:

- to receive the best treatment and care for their respective conditions.
- to be provided with rehabilitation facilities to make the best use of available skills to adjust to the conditions of living outside hospital.
- to be treated and cared for by those who are knowledgeable in the art of psychiatric healing in accordance with current acceptable ethical and standard clinical practice.
- not to have their freedom restricted unnecessarily.

- to be accepted as a partner in the treatment process.
- to be educated and provided with relevant information on their mental illness, and what to expect from treatment.
- to have family members involved in the treatment process.
- to get protection from harm, injury, and neglect.
- to be accorded human dignity, autonomy and personal individuality.
- to be informed and advised about the nature and purpose of clinical assessments, investigations and procedures to be under-taken on them. When this is not possible, the family must be informed and advised in the interests and welfare of the patient in good time.
- to confidentiality.
- to personal autonomy and integrity when requested to participate in research.
- to gain access to socials services, whether in hospital or in the community.
- to be provided with legal representation at public cost, should the need arise.
- to receive health and social care that is appropriate to his/her health needs, and in accordance with his/her relevant cultural situation.

Health worker-patient relationships

Appropriate trusting health worker-patient relationship is the basis of good clinical practice in psychiatry. This is particularly so as the psychiatric patient is often conveyed for treatment against his/her will and is thus quite vulnerable to exploitation in the course of treatment. In the Ugandan situation health workers are still viewed with respect and invested with overwhelming power and authority. Good clinical practice demands that you make every effort to bring yourself to the level of the patient and his/her carers to promote the establishment of trusting relationships. Do not use titles such as **Doctor or Professor** while introducing yourself as this has the effect of intimidating the patient into submission and or block effective communication with the patient and or carer. Remember that the patient and carer both know your title and there is no need to remind them about your professional position in society.

1. Keep making promises to patients to a minimum. Remember that it may prove difficult for you to keep such promises.
2. Set clear terms and limits to your inter-personal relationships with patients and their families. Avoid establishing clinical relationships with patients for personal financial or other gains.
3. Respect the autonomy of patients and their families.
4. Avoid patronising the patient and family.
5. Acknowledge and respect the views of patients and their families on clinical matters, and explain, where possible, that it might not be possible for you to fulfil their wishes if this is likely to clash with professional principles and or procedure.
6. Avoid taking advantage of the vulnerability of patients.
7. Always involve patients in the clinical decision-making process as far as is practicable, and obtain their valid consent to any proposed treatment. (Royal College of Psychiatrists, 2000)
8. Where the patient is unable to give consent, ensure that any treatment provided is the most appropriate for the patient and in his/her best interest. Where feasible, get the consent of the significant other for the provision of such care after explaining as fully as possible what is involved in the treatment concerned.
9. Let patients or their carers know that you acknowledge and respect the views and integrity of professional colleagues.
10. Inform the patient as far as is feasible that information you learn about them will be kept confidential.
11. Attend to patients in private unless the patient wishes to be attended to in the company of significant others, except when the patient is a child or when the presence of a significant other is considered to be essential for therapeutic or ethical reasons. This exception to the rule is particularly useful when attending to patients with a paranoid condition.

12. Avoid being a hero in your clinical practice. You may not have all the answers to a patient's problems. Where necessary acknowledge your limitations with honesty.
13. Respect the right of patients and carers to second opinion.
14. Respect the right of the patient and carer to a full explanation on diagnosis, medical procedures, treatment, treatment outcome, and likely treatment complications.
15. Answer the queries of patients and carers honestly.

Confidentiality

Under ordinary circumstances all information provided to you is privileged and must not be given to third party. However, a given psychiatric disorder may pose a danger to family members, members of the general public, or property. Psychiatric practice may meet with conflicting demands including public safety, the need to involve family and carers in developing and providing care, and the need to share information with colleagues, the police, the courts, and probation and welfare office which deals with the protection and safety of children. Not uncommonly the psychiatric patient may include the identified patient with psychiatric symptoms and the family. The needs of the identified patient may thus get muddled up with those of the family or other third, thus party complicating issues for confidentiality.

- Treat all information given to you by patient and family as confidential.
- Be familiar with the laws and regulations governing the care of the mentally ill, the protection of minors, the care and rights of suspected mentally ill prisoners and of individuals awaiting trial for various offences.
- Communicate highly accurate information to professional colleagues for the purpose of aiding colleagues in providing care to the patient.
- Where necessary, get the consent of the patient and carer before you provide information about them. Where in doubt consult

with other psychiatrists and or obtain the guidance of the Uganda Medical and Dental Practitioners' Council.

- When public safety is threatened, communicate this information to carers, the police or other health care providers after having notified the patient concerned of your intention to do so, explaining to the patient the reasons fully. Keep a record of the reasons and clinical basis for your judgement and decision to inform those concerned.
- Use confidential information for research and audit purpose according to guidelines governing research in Uganda.
- When you communicate information to doctors other than psychiatrists, this will have been done on the assumption that the information will be kept confidential and used only in providing good quality health care for the patient.
- Regularly update your knowledge of the guidance of the Uganda Medical and Dental Practitioners' Council on issues of confidentiality.

Relating to the carer

Mental illness has devastating effects on families in terms of stigmatisation, negative psychological effects, heavy economic burden in terms of care provision and or loss of income resulting from the loss of employment or from man-hours lost due to illness episodes. The disruptive social effects on family life, and the strain on emotional reserves can be severe. The outcome of mental illness is equally dependent on the way family members respond to the patient. In relating to the carer in the course of providing care to the mentally sick it is recommended that the following guidelines be followed.

1. Relate to the carer as an ally in clinical care provision.
2. Respect the views of the carer concerning clinical care. The role of the health care worker should be to provide information, advice and therapy while respecting the socio-cultural values of the patient and family.

3. Value the observation reports of the carer during outpatient reviews.

4. Support the carer in his/her efforts to cope with the care of the sick member in his/her family.

5. Keenly observe the carer for possible signs of emotional decomposition or potential sources of aggravating and/or perpetuating factors in the illness process.

6. Encourage the carer to talk about himself or herself within the context of the patient's clinical care.

7. When necessary let the carer know that you might wish to involve him/her in therapy in the course of clinical care for purposes of achieving effective clinical care outcome.

8. Offer an occasional word of praise and encouragement for the contribution of the carer.

9. Be available to the carer for impromptu consultations in times of crises.

10. Provide information on the patient's condition and educate the carer on how to recognise illness relapse, and how to maximise the patient's compliance with medical advice.

Guiding Principles

The experience of mental illness is extremely painful and distressing for both patient and family. To bring about rapid relief of distress and quick recovery, expeditious steps should be taken to provide appropriate care without causing extra pain to the patient and family. Ensure that your practice is governed by the following guidelines.

1. Keep abreast with current knowledge and practice in psychiatry and health care practice through continuing self-education.

2. Base all clinical decisions on the bio-psycho-social model of psychiatric care so as to provide and or facilitate the provision of comprehensive and holistic care for patient.

3. Regularly update your knowledge of the common aetiologies of mental illness in the community where you practice.
4. Regularly update the list of appropriate and relevant laboratory and psychosocial investigations to aid the process of diagnosis and management formulation.
5. Regularly update the list of the available facilities, and agencies with which to network in the effective, holistic and comprehensive care of the mentally sick.
6. Update, from time to time, the list of drugs available for use in the treatment of psychiatric disorders in Uganda.
7. Be aware of your own limitations and refer difficult problems, or other clinical problems with which you are not familiar to colleagues early.
8. Always work in close liaison with professional colleagues in other specialties.
9. Keep abreast with changes in the law and policies affecting the care of the sick.
10. Regularly update your knowledge of crimes committable against the mentally sick.
11. Provide psychiatric care within a dignified and humane atmosphere.
12. At all times ensure that the environment within which psychiatric care is provided does not promote self-destructive behaviour among the mentally sick.
13. Always keep in place measures to protect patients and staff from harm by dangerous patients.
14. Avoid providing care without personally assessing every patient first.
15. Constantly weigh the interests of the patients against the competing interests of families or other members of the community with whom the patients normally interact.
16. Treat patients, their families and professional colleagues with respect.

SECTION II
Selected Mental Disorders and Syndromes

4
Causes of Mental Illness

SAMUEL MALING

The causes of mental illness are often multifactorial. For example, a 30 year old woman with a positive family history of mental illness and married to a polygamous man, and who used contraceptive pills developed severe major depressive disorder with suicidal feelings. In another instance a middle-aged woman who voluntarily retired from her job invested her retirement package into a business. At the same time the woman underwent hysterectomy for persistent heavy menses associated with multiple fibroids; and her business collapsed as an additional stressor. The woman developed recurrent major depressive illness. A female student who was about to complete professional training developed severe sudden mental illness after criminal abortion complicated by heavy bleeding.

Mental illness may arise in people with a family history of the condition when they develop an infection (e.g. HIV infection or typhoid fever), or drink alcohol heavily, are exposed to war conditions or harsh domestic conditions like constant fights, experience the death of a very close relative or face the possibility of family break-up. However, at other times there may not be any link between the experience of mental illness and family history of mental illness.

In general the causes of mental illness may be grouped into the following three broad categories:

a) Intrinsic factors

b) Extrinsic environmental factors

c) The daily ups and downs (negative life events in one's social economic) of life

Internal (Intrinsic) factors

Intrinsic factors are those which the individual is born with and are related to one's genetic make-up and familial background. Note however, that people do not inherit mental illness; rather people are born with the potential to suffer from mental illness if a sufficient number of causative factors from the three classes indicated above act together at the same time or in sufficient force.

Heredity

Heredity refers to the specific genetic composition of individuals. Genes are important in life because they control all activities that humans are capable of, as well as being behind the character and lifestyles of all persons. Some mental illnesses are passed on from parent to offspring or from grand-parent to grand-children (along family line).

Chemical Substances

In the brain, there are chemical substances known as neurotransmitters (chemical messengers that work pretty like office messengers), which control human behaviour. In some cases, there may be under production or overproduction of the substances resulting into abnormal behaviour. Hormones are a special group of chemical substances that control the way the body uses its various products of digestion that are taken up in the body to support life. For instance an under production or faulty functioning of the hormone, thyroxin, may lead to depression or retarded intellectual functioning in adults and cretinism in children, while over activity leads to the experience of delusions and hallucinations in adults.

Personality

Personality refers to the characteristics that differentiate him/her from others. The physical and psychological make-up of an individual may make one liable to certain mental disorders. For instance, a person who is quiet, emotionally cold and prefers to live alone is likely to become ill with severe mental illness such as schizophrenia. A person who is outgoing, relates freely with other people and easily makes friends, and is emotionally warm but has sudden and unpredictable mood changes is likely to become ill with manic-depressive illness. An individual who worries a lot and continually doubts him/herself may suffer from depression while someone who exhibits signs of insecurity and fear may suffer from anxiety.

Aging

Degeneration of brain tissues as a result of the aging process may contribute to some mental disorders such as senile dementia.

External (Extrinsic) Environmental Factors

Extrinsic factors comprise of all acquired causes of physical ill-health that may result in the experience of mental illness, and they range from physical injury, infection to tumors. Examples of these are provided below.

- Infections such as HIV/AIDS, sleeping sickness, meningitis, typhoid fever, and brain abscesses.
- Brain trauma such as injury due to accident, or childbirth.
- Excessive and/or prolonged consumption of alcohol and habit forming drugs such as marijuana, bhangi, cocaine, pethedine, and morphine Valium etc.
- Abnormal growth in the brain (tumor)
- Malnutrition: inadequate feeding due to poverty or harmful cultural practices may deprive the brain of young children of essential nourishment thereby interfering with the optimal growth and development of the children.

Negative life events

Also known as psychosocial stressors, adverse or stressful life experiences often affect our feelings, way of thinking and interaction with people. These events are important for mental health and social wellbeing because their occurrence may lead to individuals perceiving life as meaningless, and feeling abandoned, insecure, shameful, depressed and even suicidal. Negative life events may take on every imaginable form. Some of these events may be harmless and lead to personal growth when they occur but they may lead to total confusion in other people, even though the events are relatively minor and not sufficient to interfere the persuit of life's goals. For the sake of simplicity negative life events may be grouped into the following four categories.

Loss

Bereavement, loss of social network through death, separation or moving house, loss of job, loss of property.

Disputes

Chronic disputes within the family associated with domestic violence, isolation, rejection, or discrimination or leading to marital failure, man-made disasters (e.g. war, armed conflict).

Poverty

Unemployment

Change in role status

Transition from one life stage into the next: e.g. from single marital status to married status; from being a child to being an heir; from being childless to being a parent; or from being an employee to being a director in one's institution or organisation.

Conclusion

The general causes may be summarised as follows:

- Genetic factor: positive family history of mental illness
- Infection: HIV infection, tuberculosis, typhoid fever, trypanosomiasis, meningitis
- Trauma to the head with or without obvious injury to the brain
- Cancer
- Nutritional deficiency associated with poverty, famine, pregnancy, lactation, alcohol dependence, and or following operations involving the intestines.
- Metabolic disorder: diabetes mellitus, hypoxia
- Endocrine disorder: thyroid deficiency
- Medication: e.g. contraceptive pill, aldomet, declinax, ismelin, anti-tuberculosis drug iproniazid, steroid medication
- Iatrogenic, meaning that the mental health problem has arisen as a result of treatment provided by the doctor for another

condition. For instance a fifty-five year old man who used to receive a lot of attention from his three wives and other relatives developed severe depression and died after three months of surgery for hydrocele. Following the operation the man was expected to assume responsibility for his family and lost all the social support that he previously enjoyed resulting in the depressive illness.

- Stressful life events: loss of job, bereavement, poverty, divorce or separation

Key point

Mental illness may be caused by a physical illness which must be identified and treated to achieve cure for the mental disorder. Put the other way, it is likely that some one with mental illness is suffering from physical illness, which might be the cause of the mental disorder, and that physical condition must be treated. When in doubt refer early to a senior colleague.

5
Classification of Mental Disorders

EMILIO OVUGA

Introduction

Classification in psychiatry is the grouping of related symptoms into the same category to enhance communication, clinical management, and the process of monitoring the process of recovery and clinical outcome. Functional psychiatric disorders do not arise secondary to physical illness or alcohol and substance abuse. Organic disorders on the other hand are caused by physical illness or alcohol abuse or the abuse of habit forming substances such as tobacco, marijuana and khat. The list provided is not exhaustive but indicates the types of mental disorders that are prevalent in the community.

Table 5.1: Types of Mental Disorders

Psychosis	Alcohol /Substance Disorder	Personality Disorder
• Schizophrenia	• Dependence	• Paranoid Personality Disorder
• Mania	• Abuse	• Antisocial Personality Disorder
• Depressive psychosis		• Histrionic Personality Disorder
• Paranoid state		• Schizoid Personality Disorder
• Delusional state		• Dependent Personality Disorder
• Postpartum psychosis		• Narcissistic Personality Disorder
		• Borderline Personality Disorder
		• Narcissistic Personality Disorder

Anxiety disorders	**Psychosomatic disorders**
• Generalise Anxiety disorder • Panic disorder • Obsessive-compulsive disorder • Phobia • Posttraumatic stress disorder	• Asthma • Arthritis • Dermatitis • Eczema • Essential Hypertension • Peptic ulcer disease
Organic mental disorders	**Childhood disorders**
• Delirium • Dementia • Paranoid disorder • Korsakoff's psychosis	• Behavioural disorders • Emotional disorder • Learning disability • Hyperkinetic syndrome • Disintegrative psychoses • Late onset psychosis

6
General Symptoms of Mental Disorders

EMILIO OVUGA

Introduction

Most people who suffer from mental illness may show no obvious signs of the condition even though they may experience a great deal of pain internally. There is however a small minority of individuals whose mental illness is obvious to everyone on account of their behaviour and in the way they present themselves in public. This chapter presents the signs and symptoms of mental illness in:

a) People who appear normal but suffer silently

b) People whose illness is obvious

Symptoms are more likely to indicate the need for treatment and should be taken seriously by family and friends if they are persistent, the person has mentioned them to someone or family member and they interfere with the expected day to day activities of the individual within his/her social network. Remember that many symptoms of mental illness are exaggerations of normal patterns of behaviour in daily life.

Before a detailed presentation of the general signs and symptoms is provided, basic definitions are presented below; namely of: mental health, mental illness, mental health problem, and mental disorder.

Basic concepts of mental health

Mental health

State of psychological, social, cultural, spiritual, and physical wellbeing that enables an individual to think, feel and perceive, relate and adapt to his or her environment, and to function and make personal choices optimally in the social and economic environment. General Symptoms of Mental Disorders

Mental disorder
A specific diagnosis of a condition or type of mental illness that is made by a trained mental health professional after formal psychiatric assessment or interview.

Mental health problem
Specific social, personal or psychological problems that an individual experiences as a result of mental illness.

General signs and symptoms of mental illness in a person who appears normal

- Unexplained body aches and pains
- Palpitations, persistent or recurrent headache
- Vague general ill health which does not go away on treatment
- Change in pattern of behaviour including change in social habits, which may be gradual in onset and develops over time
- Lack of regard for self-care; becoming shabby in appearance
- Loss of interest in gainful social or economic activity

Symptoms and signs in people with obvious mental illness

The signs and symptoms of mental illness are described under the following categories:

- Speech
- Thought
- Emotion or mood
- Perception
- Cognition
- Intellect
- Personality
- Appearance and behaviour

Speech

Speech is the way we put together our thoughts in words, either orally or in writing. Our speech tells other people about our inner world. Disorder of speech may take any of the following forms.

- ***Muteness*** refers to the absence of speech as in severe depression, severe schizophrenia or disease of the brain stem (midbrain).
- ***Pressure of speech*** refers to the tendency to say as much as one can within the same unit time as in mania.
- ***Incoherence of speech*** refers to the lack of logical order and relationships between ideas in what the patient says as in schizophrenia.
- ***Poverty of content of speech*** refers to lack of substance in what a person says; the individual says much but it is difficult to recognise the real ideas that he/she is trying to convey
- ***Circumstantiality in speech*** refers to a pattern of speech in which a person goes round an idea in circles before he/she finally makes the point directly

Thinking

Thinking is the ability to process information in ones mind in both content and form and organise it for expression or communication to others in through speech or other form of behaviour. Disorders of thinking occur in the following forms.

a) Stream of thought

b) Form of thought

c) Content of thought

a) **Stream of thought** refers to the way ideas flow as expressed in speech.

   - ***Pressure of thought*** refers to the abundance and varied expression of ideas as in mania.
   - ***Flight of ideas*** refers to rapid flow and expression of ideas within the same unit time with rapid shift from one idea to another.
   - ***Poverty of thought*** refers to thoughts and ideas that are scarce and the individual uses few words
   - ***Thought block*** refers to the experience of the patient characterised by sudden blankness and or emptiness, and the patient loses track of his/her own thoughts.

b) **Form of thought** refers to how ideas are connected and related to each other. The following are the disorders of form of formal thought. Note that thinking may become confused in normal people who are tired, or who have taken drugs such as sleeping pills or alcohol.

- ***Loosening of association*** refers to lack of connection between ideas as occurs in schizophrenia.
- ***Perseveration*** refers to repetitive utterance of the same words irrespective of the nature of question or nature of conversation as occurs in acute organic mental disorder.
- ***Echolalia*** is the repetition by the individual of what the doctor or another person has said, just like a child who is learning to acquire speech repeats what an adult says to the child. Echolalia occurs in severe learning disability or schizophrenia.

c) **Content of thought** refers to the quality of message being transmitted. Several forms of disorder of content of thought are frequently encountered in clinical work with patients.

  - ***Delusions*** are false beliefs or convictions that cannot be changed by rational arguments or evidence to the contrary, and are not shared by people from the same social cultural and religious background and experience.
  - ***Derealisation*** refers to the experience that everything in the surrounding seems to have changed and is strange. This experience may occur in schizophrenia, depressive illness, during fatigue or severe physical illness, as part of an epileptic attack or during an attack of migraine headache.
  - ***Depersonalisation*** refers to the patient's experience that he or she seems to have changed; that some part of his or body looks different in size, shape of texture (complexion and smoothness). This experience may occur in schizophrenia, depressive illness, and severe anxiety disorder or as part of an epileptic attack or during an attack of migraine headache. The same experience during fatigue or severe physical illness may be normal if there is no accompanying psychosis, depression or anxiety.

- ***Passivity Phenomenon*** refers to the experience in schizophrenia that his one's actions, feelings, thoughts or ideas are controlled by some foreign and mysterious agent.
- ***Thought withdrawal*** refers to the experience that one's ideas are mysteriously removed as occurs in schizophrenia. The patient may complain that his or her political enemies remove his or her ideas for their own personal ambitions.
- ***Thought broadcasting*** refers to the patient's experience that his or her ideas are being broadcasted live for other people to hear. Again the patient may attribute this experience to his or her enemies. The experience occurs in schizophrenia
- ***Running commentary*** refers to the experience in which a person hears a running commentary on his or her every action, thoughts and feelings; the experience is like hearing the commentator in a football match providing information on a football match as it is played. For example one patient complained that even when he went to the toilet, his enemies commented on his intention to go to the toilet or latrine, unfastening his belt, sitting or squatting and the very act of opening bowels, and they would then laugh at him. Another patient reported that his enemies seemed to know and say ahead of him what he intended to say even though he remained silent. Running commentaries typically occur in schizophrenia.
- ***Grandiose delusions*** refer to the belief that one is somebody great or important and occur in organic mental illness, schizophrenia or mania.
- ***Delusions of guilt and worthlessness*** refers to the patient's belief that he or she is a sinner and is not worthy to live as in severe depressive illness; this type of delusion may result in suicide or attempted suicide if not recognised early.
- ***Delusion of jealousy*** refers to person's belief that the spouse or partner is being unfaithful. This type of delusion commonly occurs in people who suffer from the effects of long history of alcohol abuse, in schizophrenia or mania.

Emotion/Mood

Mood is the sustained state of how happy or sad one feels. Mood may be *elated* and characterised by *excessive happiness* as in mania, or depressed with unusual and persistent experience of *sadness* or *unhappiness* as in depressive illness. Sometimes the patient's mood may be *irritable* characterised by easily being annoyed as in mania or depressive illness. If mood fluctuates without warning, say from extreme happiness to anger or depression and weeping, the mood is referred to as *labile mood.*

Perception

Perception is the process through which we become aware of our environment by means of the senses. There are two main types of perceptual disorders, which are *illusions* and *hallucinations*.

Illusion refers to the misinterpretation of a sensory stimulus e.g. mistaking an ant-hill at dusk for an enemy crouching low in wait; mistaking a piece of rope on the floor of one's hut as being a snake; or the singing of birds in a nearby tree as the voices of one's enemies discussing plans for effecting one's arrest.

Note that an illusion may be normal if it occurs during situations of poor sensory stimulation, such as at dusk; if the individual is fatigued mentally and physically; or if the individual is drugged with a sedative, sleeping pill or alcohol.

Hallucination refers to perception without sensory stimulus and may occur in all the sensory modalities as follows:

(i) ***Auditory hallucination*** refers to the experience of hearing voices which other people nearby do not hear. For instance an individual complained that he clearly heard enemies discuss and despise him for being a drunkard and sinner, but who other people around could not hear.

(ii) ***Visual hallucination*** refers to the experience of seeing objects, which do not exist. For example a patient may arm him with a stick and attack enemies that he herself sees but who by-standers cannot see. For instance a patient who saw very many tiny green people coming to attack him as a result of intoxication with a stimulant hurled stones at them while warning by-standers to escape. Visual hallucinations may signify an acute illness due to physical condition or drug abuse, but usually occur in schizophrenia, mania or in epilepsy.

(iii) ***Tactile hallucination*** refers to the experience of sense of touch without existing stimulus i.e. insects crawling on the body as occurs in alcohol or other drug withdrawal state.

(iv) ***Olfactory hallucination*** means smelling things, which do not exist. These smells may be of heavy nauseating nature as occurs in temporal lobe epilepsy or due to the presence of a tumor pressing on the olfactory nerve.

(v) ***Gustatory hallucination*** refers the experience of strange taste in the mouth as part of an epileptic attack or due to a tumor pressing on the brain in the floor of the skull.

Intellect

Intellect refers to the ability to reason or think logically and systematically. This ability enables an individual to receive and process, interpret and use information and other forms of experience for survival and adaptation in life. Disorders of intellect typically present in the form of inability to learn, recall, remember and use new information as occurs in learning disability in children or dementia in adults.

Memory

Memory is a special aspect of intellectual functioning and refers to the ability to recall past events. Disorders of Memory are manifested in forgetfulness and inability to remember important events in a person's life or the life of the family or community. Memory disorders can be classified as immediate, short and long term.

- ***Disorder of immediate memory*** refers to the inability to remember events that have just occurred as when one asks an individual to fails to correctly recite information immediately after he or she has been given.
- ***Disorder of short-term memory*** refers to a person's inability to remember events that happened within a period of up to 15 minutes
- ***Disorder of long-term memory*** refers to a person's inability to recall of events that occurred long time ago, for instance when a person is asked

to report the details of an event that he/she experienced five years ago or fails to correctly give the ages or birthdates of his/her children.

Note that performance on clinical tests of memory may be poor if an individual is fatigued or is heavily sedated.

Motor Function

Motor function comprises of movements, facial expression, posturing and mannerisms. Disorder of motor function may manifest in the following ways.

- Restlessness
- Overactivity
- Slowness
- Abnormal posturing and positioning
- Mannerism, twitches, grimacing, shrugging of the shoulders, purposeless movement of the arms, etc

Consciousness

Consciousness refers to the state of an individual being awareness of the environment. Disorders of consciousness may vary from mild to severe impairment; i.e. from a state of being drowsy to being deeply unconscious. Suspicion of disordered consciousness should lead to suspicion of a severe physical condition being responsible for a given mental health problem, e.g. liver or renal failure, hyperglycemia in diabetes mellitus, overdose with insulin or other hypoglycemic medication, intoxication with a sedative drug or alcohol overdose, intracranial infection, or intracranial tumor such as Subdural hematoma, or head injury.

Cognition

Cognition is a special form of consciousness and refers to the status of being knowledgeable about the environment. Tests of cognition (listed below) are used to test whether an individual suffers from a mental disorder that may be caused by a condition that affects the functioning of the brain and is probably responsible for the mental disorder.

- Disorder of attention
- Disorder of concentration
- Orientation
- Memory
- Level of consciousness

Attention refers to the ability of an individual to focus his or mind to a task till that task is completed. Disorder of attention may manifest in an individual who responds to almost every trivial stimulus. For a person who suffers from delirium due to sleeping sickness by responding to foot-steps, rustle of paper, clanging of plates in the course of clinical interview. In this case the disorder of attention is termed *short attention span*. A person with short attention span will fail to learn new information, and therefore will have poor immediate and short-term memories.

Disorder of concentration, referred to as *impaired concentration,* refers to the inability of an individual to apply his/her mind to one task till that task is completed. This disorder may manifest in the individual being fatigued in the course of the exercise and abandoning the task. The standard test for concentration is to ask an individual to perform a series of sub-tractions of seven from numbers beginning with 100. The expected result should be correct answers at every stage with the exercise taking a maximum of 2 and half to 3 minutes.

Orientation refers to a state in which an individual correctly tells the time of day, the place he/she is in and correctly identifies the people in his/her vicinity. Organic mental disorders may lead to *poor orientation* to time, place and or person. For example the clinical interview room may be described as a market place and the time of day as 9.00 o'clock in the evening.

Disorders of memory, as defined earlier may be of three types; namely: immediate, short-term and long-term. (See section on memory)

Level of consciousness may vary from *lethargy, drowsiness, sleepiness, stupor,* to *coma*. The individual's level of being in contact with the surroundings may therefore fluctuate according to the level of consciousness; he/she may be easily awakened from being lethargic, drowsy or sleepy but soon slips back into the status. Note that occasionally individuals who suffer from stroke involving the mid-brain may not seem to be in coma as they appear fully awake and follow the health care provider around the bed. This type of coma is referred to as *coma vigil* and is severe in form. The level of consciousness may be tested for by applying various levels of pressure to the sternum or forehead, or calling the individual by name.

Relationship

Relationship is the way in which we interact with other people around us. The Disorders of relationship are as follows:

- Social withdrawal
- Poor interpersonal relations
- Over-familiarity

Sleep Disorders

Sleep disorders are among the commonest problems that patients present with, whether they have physical illness or psychiatric disorder. The disorders may assume one of three forms. Physical conditions associated with pain, depression, anxiety and acute psychosocial problems in daily life are the commonest causes of disturbed sleep.

- Failure to fall asleep in early hours of night suggests the presence of acute or chronic psychosocial problems associated with worries.
- Failure to sleep in late hours or the night, associated with early wakening is usually associated with severe depressive illness.
- Interrupted sleep, associated with frightening dreams may be due to anxiety or depressive illness. Acute Schizophrenia and alcohol withdrawal state or delirium with severe auditory and visual hallucinations may also be responsible for interrupted sleep throughout the night.

7
Depression

EMILIO OVUGA

Prevalence

Overall 15-42% of different population groups in Uganda suffer from depressive illness (Orley, 1979; Ovuga et al, 2005). In Uganda the prevalence of depression has been shown to vary from region to region, and according to educational level (Ovuga et al, 2005). Elsewhere the prevalence of depression has been shown to vary from country to country and even within the same country (Weissman et al, 1996).

In general expect to diagnose depression-requiring treatment in one out of every 5 to 10 patients attending primary care. You should expect to see more people with depression among the rural poor, among those with low education and among individuals who have experienced a significant psychosocial stressor in the past three months.

Help-seeking behaviour

However 5-30% of individuals with depression get treatment for their condition even when the services are available to them (Ovuga, 2005) suggesting that personal, social and cultural factors probably determine care seeking behaviour.

Aetiology

Depression in Uganda is related to poverty, adverse interpersonal relationships, loss or bereavement, physical illness including infection with HIV. Forty percent of cases of depression co-exist with alcohol dependence, and 20%, anxiety disorder.

Depression may be primary or due to:

- Another psychiatric disorder, e.g. schizophrenia.
- A general medical illness, e.g. hypothyroidism, cancer, hypertension.
- Medication, e.g. steroid therapy, methyldopa.
- The abuse of substance of abuse, e.g. alcohol.

Features of depression

- Lack of sleep or disturbed sleep as a result of nightmares
- Unexplained sadness or unhappiness (almost whole day) for at least 2 weeks.
- Loss of interest for social contact (wants to be alone).
- Loss of interest in usual pleasurable activities (has no interest in doing anything at all that used to be of interest).
- Loss of capacity for happiness (does not know happiness, joy, enjoyment).
- Poor or excessive sleep.
- Poor or excessive appetite for food.
- Numerous body complaints.
- Lack of energy (has unexplained general weakness)
- Difficulty carrying out usual work (everything is needs extra effort and energy to carry out).
- Too much worrying or thinking (about personal problems).
- Absent-mindedness, poor concentration, poor memory (has to constantly remind self in order to remember things; may keep diary of what everyday in order not to forget).
- Excessive worries over the future (fears to face the future; tomorrow seems to heavy a burden to carry; worries as to how he/she will go through each day that comes)
- Fear of dying, recurrent death wishes or suicidal thoughts (including the wish to get killed by someone in a fight; wish to be run over by a motor vehicle).
- Low self-esteem - ideas of worthlessness, failure, guilt, self-blame; compares self with "successful" peers and may regret and complain about missed opportunities.
- Lacking courage and self-confidence; postpones plans only to regret it later.

Depression may present with psychotic features:

- Delusions: belief, for example, that one is responsible for all the suffering in the world and therefore should be punished for all the sins in the world; believing that one is so worthless that one is not fit to be cared for.
- Hallucinations: hearing one's grand-children crying as they are tortured by one's enemies.
- Loss of insight: lacking the ability to recognise that one needs help for one's condition.

Depression may co-exist and present with anxiety:

- Unexplained fear or fear that is inappropriate for the individual
- Experience of inability to feel relaxed; feeling tense and uneasy
- Expecting doom, tragedy, bad news
- Episodes of panic in which the individual experience intense fear associated with panic, nervousness, strong urge for micturition or to open bowels, sweating, tremors, and restlessness

Making diagnosis of depression

Detect depression with clinical interview; depression is very common in the community. Have a high index of suspicion for depression; 1 in 10 adults at a health unit may be depressed and may require antidepressant medication. If any adult answers "Yes" to the first question below and a further "Yes" to any one other question, he/she probably will benefit from antidepressant medication. Ask directly for the features of depression, for example:

1. Have you been feeling sad or unhappy over the past 2 to 4 weeks?
2. If so have you been able to enjoy anything at all, such as being with family, friends, or participating in activities that you normally enjoy doing at home or place of work?
3. Are you any more interested in doing the things you normally do?
4. Have you experienced the problems of absent-mindedness and/or forgetfulness; are you troubled by the problem of misplacing items and failing to find them for some time or having to write things down to make sure you do not forget them?

5. If so have you been feeling that it would be better if you were dead than alive?

Principles of Management of Depression:

- Develop treatment plan with the patient and carer.
- Ascertain that the depression is not due to a general medical condition, medication or substance abuse.

Educate the patient and carer about depression:

- Depression is a medical illness.
- Effective treatment is available.
- Treatment leads to complete symptom resolution.
- There are several treatment options (list them).
- The condition tends to recur (50% chance after the first episode; 70% after a second episode; 90% after a third episode; 100% after third and subsequent episodes); adequate treatment for at least 6 months on daily dose of the recommended medication is required to prevent the condition becoming chronic.
- Patience and persistence to comply with medical advice is useful to maintain good health.
- Treatment for any medical condition if detected is essential in addition to treating the depression itself; that it might become necessary to refer to the physician or other health care specialist as the need arises.
- An offending medication may be discontinued if the depression is due to that medication.
- Use of electro-convulsive therapy may be considered if there is no clinical progress within four weeks on adequate dose of antidepressant medication.
- Once appropriate antidepressant medication has been started this must be continued uninterrupted for 6-8 months.
- During the course of antidepressant medication the patient should preferably not take alcoholic beverages.
- Assess clinical progress regularly.

- Let the patient know that you understand his/her situation.
- If there is a risk of suicide advise for hospitalisation; or tell the patient that the relatives should know about his/her feelings; and enter into a contract to assure that the patient will communicate any future suicidal urges immediately to the nearest relative or other trusted person.
- Inform the patient and carer that you might refer him/her to a senior colleague as necessary. (Note that the patients and carers in our setting regard health facilities as one-stop unit where their problems should be settled by only one health worker and they might resent the idea of referral).

Treatment options

There are three main approaches to the treatment of depression.

1. Medication, e.g. Imipramine
2. Psychological, e.g. simple counselling, interpersonal therapy, cognitive therapy, and cognitive-behaviour therapy. Training in the provision of these psychotherapeutic services is needed; e.g. helping a woman get over three consecutive deaths of her children before their 10th birthday.
3. Social management: Rehabilitation to help the patient stay at the place of work or resume usual activities of daily living in the community; involvement of the family in modifying harmful social factors such as discussing causes and avenues for overcoming disputes; helping someone overcome economic hardships.

Drugs

The drugs recommended at district level are

- Antidepressants:
- Amitryptiline or Imipramine 50 mg at night and step up the dose as necessary. You need to wait for 2 – 3 weeks before signs of recovery can be seen. For children aged 10-16 years the starting dose of these antidepressant drugs is 25 mg.
- Newer antidepressant drugs known as SSRIs (e.g. Fluoxetine, Paroxetine) are available on the open market and they act faster but are not yet official

national drugs list and are therefore out of reach of the rural peasant farmer.

- Counselling

Precautions

- Person with heart disease should have a thorough examination before starting treatment.
- Watch out for side effects such as: Dry mouth blurred vision, irregular heartbeats and light-headedness or dizziness especially when the person gets out of bed

Prognosis

Most cases of depression resolve completely on treatment. A few cases of depression are complicated by anxiety disorder and or psychotic features while others become resistant to treatment due to late treatment, inappropriate initial treatment or inadequate medication with antidepressant. Depression tends to become more frequent and harder to control with advancing age of the patient; depression in younger patients should therefore be treated vigorously to limit the potential to become chronic or resistant. Medical conditions such as epilepsy, HIV/AIDS, tuberculosis, cancer, thyroid deficiency, and diabetes mellitus may be associated with depression and effectiveness of their treatment will determine the prognosis of depression. 3-4% of people with depression may commit suicide.

8
Mania

HARRIET BIRABWA

Mania is a disorder of mood (feeling state) characterised by sustained elevated happy or irritable mood. Mania is one of the commonest causes of psychiatric admission in Uganda. However symptoms of mania may also be caused by a variety of other conditions in Uganda including HIV/AIDS, alcohol and substance abuse, nutritional disturbances, hypertension and other physical conditions commonly seen in primary care.

Prevalence

Mania is estimated to affect 1-2% of the general population. In Uganda, mania is one of the leading diagnoses among people who receive in-patient care. This is because the condition presents acutely, is associated with considerable potential for the disruption of social order and therefore presents adequate grounds for urgent admission to hospital for control.

Importance of Mania

Mania is socially disruptive, predisposes to alcohol and substance abuse and crime or sexual over-involvement, and predisposes the individual to sexually transmitted illnesses. Note though that there are individuals in the general population with less severe forms of the condition, and who run successful businesses or public offices. It may therefore be difficult to differentiate such persons from members of the general population if their behaviour does not lead to grounds to suspect anything the matter with them.

Features and Diagnosis

According to the fourth edition of DSM-IV (APA, 1992), a diagnosis of mania is made on the basis of the following clinical features.

- Abnormal and persistently elevated, happy, irritable, expansive mood for at least one week.
- The additional presence of at least three of the following features

- Grandiosity and elevated self-image, e.g. one is a special person chosen by God to save the world from AIDS
- Decreased need for sleep or food, believing that time spent for these activities may be a waste of time
- More talking than usual, e.g. talking non-stop for hours; talking fast and loudly; pressured speech characterised by the individual wishing to say as much as possible within the same unit of time.
- Flight of ideas; rapidly skipping from one topic to the other during talking
- Being distractible; attention shifting from stimulus to stimulus
- Over-activity
- Excessive involvement in pleasurable activities.
- Excessive generosity; not wishing to see people miserable, and being ready to share whatever little the individual might have.

- Associated impairment in social occupational functioning
- Symptoms are not due to physical illness, or alcohol and drug abuse.

Principles of Management

Management of mania comprises of three strategies, namely; medication, social therapy, and supportive psychotherapy aimed to shorten the duration of active illness, prolong illness-free duration, reduce the number of relapses and enhance self-reliance through gainful socio-economic functioning. See section on drug therapy. The general management principles are the same as in schizophrenia.

The serious damage, which a patient with mania may cause to him/herself or to the family, requires that patients with mania should be hospitalised if their condition is seen to be severe. Antipsychotic medication is the cornerstone of treatment of mania. High doses may be required in a highly aroused, very over talkative patient.

Dosage: Chlorpromazine (Largactil) 100-300 mg 2–3 times a day. And increase the dose as necessary up to 600 mg a/day.

OR:

Haloperidol if available is the drug of choice in dose 5-10 mg 2-3 times a day; increase dose if necessary, up to 60 mg/daily in three divided doses. Watch for side effects

- Stiffness of muscles especially neck
- Drooling saliva
- Rolling the eyes to the back of head
- Skin rash
- Tongue protrusion
- Give Artane 2–5 mg once daily if side effects appear

Control of Recurrent Episodes

If three or more episodes occur in 12 months, it is advisable to use the anti-convulsant drug Carbamazepine (tegretol) in the dose of 200-400 mg twice daily. Success will depend on the extent to which the patient understands and appreciates the negative impact of his or her condition on his or her life and that of the family or the community. The patient who has had two episodes of mania may be aware of the signs of relapse; such as total lack of sleep, excessive happiness, and decreased need to rest. Use this understanding as a basis to motivate him or her to remain on medication. However it may be difficult for the patient to recognise the onset of relapse, and this fact should be used to request the patient to allow family or trusted friends to seek medical attention for him/her in case the patient lacks capacity to seek treatment personally.

Prognosis

One in every three patients with mania becomes chronic and will require medication in the long-term. In a small proportion of patients, a manic episode is preceded or followed by a depressive disorder episode, thus giving rise to the name, *bipolar affective disorder* or *manic-depressive psychosis*. Sometimes patients with mania or depression may swing from one condition to another and vice versa (*Bipolar Manic-depressive disorder*) when undergoing treatment; continuation of medication is recommended in most cases.

9
Anxiety Disorders

EMILIO OVUGA

This is a syndrome in which the Psychological and Physical symptoms are those of anxiety and which are not secondary to any physical or psychiatric illness.

Prevalence

At least 9% of the general population suffers from anxiety disorder. The following categories of anxiety disorder do affect people in Uganda; namely: Social Phobia, Obsessive-compulsive disorder, Panic disorder and Generalised Anxiety Disorder. These types of anxiety disorder are extremely painful, and socially and occupationally incapacitating. Remember that anxiety disorder is one of the leading causes of disability. Anxiety often co-exists with other types of psychiatric disorder including affective disorder and alcohol use. Many patients who suffer from physical illness also experience panic attacks, for example cancer.

Aetiology of Anxiety

In most cases the individual's previous character is an anxious one, chronically worried feeling that anything worse is going to happen even without apparent cause. Anxiety may be primary or secondary. Secondary anxiety disorder may be due to:

- Another psychiatric disorder, e.g. depression, schizophrenia.
- A general medical condition, e.g. hypertension, hyper-parathyroidism, cardiac arrhythmias, temporal lobe epilepsy, hypoglycaemia.
- Medication, e.g. excessive use of caffeine.
- Substance abuse, e.g. alcohol withdrawal

Signs and Symptoms of Generalised Anxiety

These are classified into 2:

- The Physical Symptoms and
- The Psychological Symptoms

Physical Symptoms

- Poor appetite
- Sweating
- Tremors
- Tachycardia - palpitations
- Over breathing and difficult in breathing in.
- Dry mouth
- Headache
- Frequency in micturition.
- Diarrhoea
- Nausea
- Disturbance of monthly periods

Psychological Symptoms

- Excess worry for no reason (free-floating anxiety).
- Lack of concentration
- Irritability
- Tearfulness
- Indecisiveness
- Restlessness
- Worry over physical symptoms
- Feeling dreadful (fearful of impending doom).
- Loss of libido.
- Lack of attention and concentration

Assessment

While assessing, one should endeavor to exclude the physical illness as most of the signs and symptoms of generalised anxiety may be like those of chronic physical conditions.

Management

- Supportive Counselling
- Be sympathetic and involve the family

Management

A) Medication:

- Develop treatment plan with the patient.
- Ensure that the anxiety is not due to a general medical condition, medication or illicit substance use.
- Educate the patient and carer about anxiety.
- Attend to general medical condition if detected.
- Discontinue offending medication if primary cause of anxiety.
- Choose and use an appropriate anxiolytic drug for no more than two weeks, e.g. Diazepam (5-10 mg three times daily), Chlordiazepoxide (10-20 mg twice daily). Low doses of neuroleptic medication may be used, e.g. 25-50 mg of Chlorpromazine three times per day; 2 mg of Haloperidol three times per day; and 2 mg of Trifluoperazine three times per day.
- Assess clinical progress regularly.
- Refer early if in doubt.

B) Psychotherapy

Specific forms of behavioural psychotherapy are effective for different types of anxiety disorder:

- *Muscle relaxation* (Generalised anxiety or panic disorder)
- *Breathing exercises* (Generalised anxiety or panic disorder)
- *Systematic desensitisation* (Various forms of phobia)
- *Exposure with response prevention* (obsessive-compulsive disorder)
- *Breathing into a polythene back* (panic disorder)

Prognosis

Recurrent episodes are expected in the remaining 80-90% of cases. Most patients can learn how to control the distressing symptoms of recurrent episodes of anxiety using relaxation and breathing exercises.

Key point

The use of medication with psychotherapy has better clinical outcome. Where in doubt refer to a senior colleague early. Specific training in the use of the behavioural techniques may be required for better outcome.

10
Psychosis

EMILIO OVUGA

Prevalence

Psychosis affects 1-2% of the general population.

Features

Detect psychosis with clinical interview. Ask directly for the features of psychosis.

- Delusions.
- Hallucinations.
- Bizarre, violent and irrational behaviour

Aetiology

1. Psychosis may be primary or secondary; primary psychosis has no demonstrable cause and is also known as functional psychosis.
2. Secondary psychosis may be due to:
   - General physical illness, e.g. HIV/AIDS, typhoid, hypertension.
   - Medication, e.g. steroid medication.
   - Substance abuse, e.g. cannabis, miraa (khat, mairungi).

Management

1. Develop treatment plan with the patient and or carer.
2. Ensure that the psychosis is not due to general medical illness, the result of medication, or due to substance abuse.
3. Start treatment with an appropriate neuroleptic.
4. Attend to offending general medical condition responsible for the psychosis.
5. Educate the patient and carer about psychotic illness.

6. Provide supportive psychotherapy.
7. Review clinical progress regularly.
8. Refer early if in doubt.

Drug treatment at district level includes one of the following options.
Chlorpromazine: 100-300 mg 1-3 times per day
Haloperidol: 5-15 mg 1-3 times per day.
Fluphenazine Decanoate injection: 25-50 mg I.M.I. once a month for maintenance.

Prognosis

Complete recovery is expected in up to 80% of cases. The course of illness in 20% is chronic. For optimal results, medication should be continued for at least 12 months in schizophrenia.

11
Schizophrenia

Emilio Ovuga

Schizophrenia is one of the severest forms of mental illness, which tend to run a chronic course. It affects 1% of the general population.

Schizophrenia is important to remember because it is common in primary care in Uganda. In fact this condition takes fourth position in frequency according to hospital statistics of Butabika hospital. Thus, schizophrenia is important because it is the most severe psychiatric disorder with a progressively deteriorating course over time. Each time a person with the condition suffers a relapse, he or she takes longer on larger doses of medication before he or she can recover from the new illness episode.

Each illness episode leaves the individual with a permanent scar on his personality; the individual almost invariably loses their ability for independent living and faces the risk of being rejected by his or her family and community. There are five main types of schizophrenia, namely: paranoid sub-type, catatonic sub-type, simple sub-type, hebephrenic sub-type, and disorganised sub-type.

Types of Schizophrenia

Paranoid schizophrenia

The main feature of the paranoid sub-type is a well-organised paranoid delusions consisting of a system of mistrust for the intentions of others, sense of personal vulnerability in the face of perceived threat from the social environment, and the belief that one is the object of an orchestrated malice and plot to frustrate or destroy. Paranoid schizophrenia is usually first diagnosed after the age of thirty-five, and is considered to hold the best prognosis.

Catatonic schizophrenia

The main feature of this sub-type is the period disturbance in motor function characterised either by excitement and violence or severe retardation and marked reduction in motor and intellectual activity.

Simple schizophrenia

This sub-type is characterised by an insidious and gradual onset of illness, taking many years for relatives and family to notice that something is really wrong. In the early stages, what are usually obvious are the oddities in behaviour, eccentricities in character and the asocial solitary lifestyle that characterise the individual in the early stages of the illness that see the individual lose their capacity for work and self-care. Simple schizophrenia is usually first occurs in late twenties or early thirties.

Hebephrenic schizophrenia

This sub-type is characterised by disorganised thinking process and content; incoherence is the main feature of the disorder. Hebephrenic schizophrenia usually first occurs in the teen years and may be responsible for poor academic performance of those affected.

Disorganised schizophrenia

This sub-type has no specific delineating feature but consists of a mixture of the features of the other four sub-types in varying proportions.

Causes of Schizophrenia

The cause of schizophrenia is a combination of factors and these include:-

- Genetic predisposition: Schizophrenia is known to run in families
- Personality: People who are withdrawn, having no friends and lead solitary lives and prefer being in isolation than in a group (schizoid personality) are more likely to suffer from schizophrenia.
- Stressful events: there are likely to precipitate a breakdown associated with schizophrenia (refer to unit I for causes of mental disorders).

Signs and symptoms

1. Personal appearance tends to be neglected and the individual ends up being dirty / filthy.
2. The patients withdraw into a world of their own.
3. Lack of interest in the environment.
4. Perception disorders: the common ones are auditory hallucinations of:-

a) third party auditory hallucinations.
b) commanding voices to which the patients are compelled to respond.
c) voices giving running commentary on the person's action.
d) tactile hallucinations may also be present

5. Lack of drive and will power.
6. Disturbances in thought include:-

a) Delusions (persecution; the belief that other people are plotting to kill, delusions of grandeur; the belief that one is special, nihilistic tendencies; the belief that one's internal organs such as the intestines have been cut into pieces or that the head is filled with gas)
b) Thought blocking (the experience that ideas suddenly stop flowing, commonly known as empty mind)
c) Thought withdrawal (ideas being taken away from the mind).
d) Thought broadcasting (the experience that one's thoughts are broadcast on radio and television for other people to hear)
e) Thought spoken out aloud (the experience that one's thoughts are spoken out loud even though one is keeping silent)
f) Thought insertion (the experience that foreign ideas are mysteriously put in one's head)
g) Passivity phenomenon (the experience that one's actions are being controlled by some mysterious force, e.g. that even when one laughs, it is not oneself who is laughing but some other agent; that a cat passes stool on one's behalf, etc)

7. Disturbances in behaviour include

a) Childish behaviour; smiling, talking, or laughing to oneself
b) Sudden violence in response to hallucinations or delusions, but rare
c) Abnormal gestures, postures, stupor.
d) Being restless, wandering aimlessly.
e) Echopraxia – repetition of actions being of the interviewer.

8. Disturbances of mood - mood may be flat, blank, blunted or inappropriate (incongruent mood - emotional incontinence)

9. Disturbance of speech

   a) Echolalia - repetition of words being said by the interviewer
   b) Incoherence and irrelevancy
   c) Neologisms/word salads

Diagnosis

Schizophrenia is a major mental disorder, which usually starts at early age. It tends to be chronic and to run a downward course. The disorder is characterised by change in personality, leading to inability to relate to others, disturbed moods, impaired perception and disrupted thought processes and will power.

A diagnosis of schizophrenia is made on the basis of the following grounds;

- Two or more of the following characteristic symptoms
  - Delusions
  - Hallucinations
  - Hallucinations
  - Disorganised incoherent speech
  - Disorganised behaviour
  - Reduced emotional response, reduced volition or speech, and reduced social contact in spite of the presence of opportunities for adequate social interaction.
- Impaired social economic functioning in spite of opportunities for adequate work.
- Duration of symptoms of one month for active symptoms and six months for non-active illness.
- The illness is not due to physical condition such as HIV/AIDS or alcohol or substance abuse.

Principles of Management of Schizophrenia

The management of schizophrenia is similar to the treatment of psychosis. However, the outcome of schizophrenia depends on the use of a combination of strategies in management, including drug therapy, social therapy, and supportive psychotherapy. In providing care to someone with probable schizophrenia, one must ensure that conditions that may appear in the same way as schizophrenia are excluded. These conditions include mania, alcohol and substance abuse, organic mental disorder and epilepsy. Hence all new patients suspected to be suffering from Schizophrenia should be referred to the district hospital for proper diagnosis and treatment. Then continue with follow up to facilitate the rehabilitation, socialization and resettlement of patients in their home communities. These activities are recommended:

- Encourage formation of support groups such as Schizophrenia Fellowships among patients and relatives
- Use of antipsychotic drugs.
- Counseling.

Prognosis

The prognosis of schizophrenia is typically poor in developed countries. However, in Uganda as in other third world countries, the outlook for schizophrenia is good. To improve outcome one needs to promote compliance, be available to provide support and answer questions from the patient and family in relation to the illness, use long acting depot medications if necessary and involve the patient and family in planning maintenance treatment. Factors associated with good outcome in schizophrenia include sudden onset, high levels of excitement, the presence of a significant psychosocial stressor, absence of previous family history of mental illness, and good prior personality of the individual.

12

Organic Mental Disorders

EMILIO OVUGA

Organic mental disorders are mental illnesses that arise due to physical illness. In routine clinical care it is advisable to think of common mental disorders in terms of the presence or absence of physical illness to ensure that pre-existing physical factors in mental illness are recognised, investigated and appropriately treated as treatment as mental disorder is provided.

Characteristics of organic mental disorder

1. Presence of physical illness and fever
2. Apathy and social withdrawal or restlessness and over activity of after onset.
3. Absent-mindedness
4. Forgetfulness or misplacement of items
5. Request for questions or instructions to be repeated
6. Cognitive impairment; these are quick short-hand signs for organic mental disorder and should be performed in all cases. Clues to their presence include absent-mindedness; forgetfulness in the course of interview; apathy or overactivity.
   a) Short attention span: inattention to the present; patient leaves tasks unfinished.
   b) Poor concentration: patient cannot perform serial-7 test
   c) Poor memory: immediate and short-term for delirium or long-term for dementia
   d) Disorientation to person, time and place
   e) Perseveration: the repetition of the same answer irrespective of what is asked

f) Apraxia: the inability to perform motor functions correctly, e.g. tracing a design, completing a drawing or describing setting, characters and actions depicted in a drawing
g) Impaired judgment: inability to explain the hidden implications in behaviour
h) Impaired abstract thinking: inability to give the correct meaning to a proverb in common usage.

Sometimes organic mental disorders may not have the above characteristics until in late stages of mental disorder, and a high index of suspicion should govern every encounter with patients.

13
Delirium

EMILIO OVUGA

Prevalence

The prevalence in the general population in Uganda is unknown.

Aetiology

Delirium is an abrupt onset of mental disorder due to any of several general medical conditions, e.g. HIV/AIDS, liver disease, renal failure, septicaemia, meningitis, etc.

Features

Detect delirium with clinical interview and cognitive assessment.

1. Disorientation to time, place, person.
2. Poor concentration, apathy, overactivity.
3. Short attention span, absent-mindedness, inability to learn new information.
4. Poor short-term memory, inability to remember or recall information.
5. Acute onset of illness.

Management

Delirium is a medical emergency and is associated with substantial mortality or long-term morbidity if improperly managed. The symptoms of delirium tend to fluctuate rapidly, being worse at night or if there are too many distractions. Delirium is best managed in a medical ward, or in close consultation with general physicians.

- Take detailed history followed by comprehensive medical examination and mental status assessment.
- Carry out relevant and appropriate biomedical investigations.

- Start appropriate medical treatment.
- Nurse in a quiet, gently lit room particularly at night when the clinical condition may worsen.
- Avoid changing nursing staff too frequently. Respond to the patient in a consistent manner.
- Attend to general health needs. Encourage plenty of fluids orally or by the intra-venous route if the patient is unable to take anything by mouth.
- Control psychotic symptoms with appropriate dose of high potency Neuroleptic such as Haloperidol in doses recommended as in psychosis.
- Provide education to patient and or carer on delirium, reassuring them of the expected quick recovery and good long-term outcome.
- Review clinical progress daily.
- Consult a physician or senior colleague at the earliest opportunity or refer early if in doubt. Continue to work in liaison with the physician even after the transfer of the patient to a medical ward to ensure appropriate control of behavioural disorder associated with the condition.

Prognosis

Complete recovery is expected if the physical condition is treated early. A minority of cases may become chronic due to delay in treatment.

14
Delirium Tremens

EMILIO OVUGA

This is an acute psychiatric disorder which develops in a person with long history of heavy alcohol abuse. The disorder starts 8-12 hours after the last drink, usually following admission to a hospital ward, lack of funds to purchase the next drink or while on a long trip without access to the next alcoholic drink. Occasionally the problem may develop consequent upon a sudden increase in the quantity of alcohol used, e.g. when at a party. The exact prevalence of delirium tremens in Uganda is unknown. However 12% of the general population in Adjumani district has been shown to suffer from alcohol dependence (Ovuga, 2005) and 5% of admissions to adult general wards in Adjumani district hospital had delirium tremens (Odendi, 2005).

Features

Delirium tremens is associated with confusion, irritability, coarse tremors, nausea, vomiting, weakness, tachycardia, elevated blood pressure, fever, sweating, hallucinations and illusions. Delirium tremens may begin with convulsions in some 5% of cases. The general features of mental state are as described for delirium. Common differential diagnoses that must be excluded for optimal clinical care outcome include meningitis and severe malaria.

Diagnosis

- Positive history of excessive alcohol consumption over a long period of time
- Recent abstinence from or heavier intake of alcohol consumed at a special social gathering or event such as a party or ceremony; abstinence might have been brought about by lack of money, an acute illness episode such as motor vehicle accident, or long-distance travel without access to alcohol.
- Low-grade fever of sudden onset
- Confusion of acute onset, worse at night

- Prominent hallucinations that may include vivid visual hallucinations, insulting and despising auditory hallucinations, and tactile hallucinations involving insects crawling on the skin or falling out of the nostrils, eyes or mouth. The individual may be seen picking objects from space or anywhere else around him or her.
- Hallucinations may be associated with persecutory delusions.
- As a result of hallucinations and or delusions the individual may be restless, fearful, combative or may flee from enemies.
- The individual may exhibit coarse tremors and when severe, he or she may fail to walk or sit unaided due to ataxia.
- Negative blood slide for malaria parasites
- Normal laboratory findings on cerebrospinal fluid

To confirm a diagnosis of delirium tremens always ask the patient and or relatives about history and pattern of alcohol use.

Management

1. Nurse the patient in a quiet, gently lit room.
2. Avoid too many changes in nursing staff.
3. Ensure plenty of fluids orally or via the intra-venous route if the patient cannot take anything by mouth.
4. Ensure adequate rest under sedation. For this purpose high potency neuroleptic such as haloperidol, and or benzodiazepine such as diazepam or Chlordiazepoxide may be used.
5. Provide multivitamins parenterally if the patient cannot take anything orally. Provide thiamine to prevent the development of Wernicke's encephalopathy.
6. Other forms of medication depend on other aspects of the clinical problem:
   - ***Seizures:*** diazepam and or an anticonvulsant such as Phenytoin or carbamazepine for a period of at least two weeks. Thereafter conduct an EEG and decide if the anticonvulsant should be continued or not. This decision will depend on other aspects of the clinical problem, such as prior history of convulsions and the EEG report.

- ***Hallucinosis:*** high potency neuroleptic. However, note the danger of chlorpromazine use in alcohol abuse or dependence, namely, liver disease. Where available use haloperidol in the low doses of 2-5 mg twice or three times daily.
- ***Fever:*** conduct biomedical investigations and provide appropriate treatment.

Prognosis

Delirium tremens is associated with a mortality rate of 10-25% if improperly managed. However complete recovery is the rule if treatment is instituted early and provided expeditiously. Delay in the recognition and adequate treatment of delirium tremens may lead to Korsakoff's psychosis, a life-long memory disorder.

15
Alcohol and Drug Abuse (Substance Abuse)

SAMUEL MALING

Substance abuse occurs when an individual has been using an habit-forming substance in excess and for a long period of time with detrimental effects on his/her physical health, social life, and psychological well being.

Substance abuse is associated with social, physical and psychological problems. According to WHO 3% of the general population suffers from substance abuse related Mental Health problems.

The following are the commonly abused substances in Uganda.

1. Alcohol (common in self-medication in depression, anxiety and early stages of psychosis, e.g. manic disorder)
2. Tobacco
3. Diazepam (as sleeping pill, common in self-medication for anxiety and depression; may be iatrogenic, that is, introduced by the doctor in the treatment of anxiety)
4. Marijuana (among laborers, students, long-distance truck drivers)
5. Khat (Mairungi) (to dampen hunger)
6. Pethidine (among health workers or patients who have been exposed to this drug after major surgery)
7. Aviation fuel, petrol, glue, thinner (among street children)
8. Cocaine (common among students from rich and or social prominent families)
9. Heroin (as for cocaine)
10. Mandrax (methaqualone) (as for diazepam)
11. Amphetamine (students, laborers, long-distance truck drivers to promote alertness and stamina)

12. Mogadon (as for diazepam)
13. Magic mushroom (youth in dance places, musicians)

The following groups are prone to use substances of abuse as indicated above.

- Medical workers (anti-anxiety drugs, hypnotics and sedatives, pethine).
- Adolescents and children of school going age from rich families (alcohol, stimulants).
- Idle, unemployed youth (cannabis, khat)
- Manual laborers (cannabis, tobacco, khat)
- People who work in breweries (various alcoholic beverages)
- Hotel workers (various alcoholic beverages)
- Taxi and long distance drivers (cannabis, khat)
- Students of higher learning institutions (stimulants, cannabis)
- Prostitutes (various alcoholic beverages, heroine, cocaine)
- Music Dance & Drama groups (ecstasy, speed)

Factors that predispose people to substance abuse:

1. Social economic stressors.
2. Cultural practices.
3. Availability of drugs of abuse
4. Peer pressure
5. Pressure to achieve
6. Broken family environment
7. Underlying mental illness e.g. depression, anxiety etc.

Stages of the process of substance abuse:-

1. **Experimentation:** Try out one, or on a few occasions- usually in the peer group.
2. **Social use:** This is when the individual uses the drug regularly.

3. **Abuse:** Is regular intoxication with a substance of abuse, which occurs out of the social context. The individual may be intoxicated during the day, may get problems at work, may have marital discord and may do what is contrary to what the law requires.

4. **Tolerance:** Is a tendency to take increased doses of the substance to get the desired effect.

5. **Dependency:** When the substance of abuse is not used at the scheduled time withdrawal symptoms occur (Physical dependency). Psychological dependence refers to the repeated psychological need for the effects offered by a substance.

Prevention of substance abuse

Prevention is best achieved by the use of support groups. In the individual case prevention begins with assessing the pattern and potential magnitude of the use of abused substance, followed by the management of the active use of the abused substance (detoxification) before involving the person in the preventive program.

Recognition of alcohol abuse (Assessment of patient using cage)

Alcohol abuse often goes undetected because subjects conceal the extent of their drinking. Doctors and other professionals often do not ask the right questions. It should be standard practice to ask all patients (medical, surgical and psychiatric) about their alcohol consumption.

The use of four key questions referred to as **CAGE** will help to identify alcohol abuse. **CAGE** is from the initial letters of the following words: **C**ut, **A**nnoyed, **G**uilty and **E**ye-opener. Ask the following.

1. Have you ever felt that you ought to **Cut down** on your drinking?

2. Have people **A**nnoyed you by criticizing your drinking habits?

3. Have you ever felt **G**uilty about your drinking?

4. Have you ever had a drink first thing in the morning (an **E**ye opener) to steady your nerves or get rid of a hangover?

Note: Two or more positive replies identify alcohol abuse and one positive reply, possible current use.

Health Education

The health care provider should educate the patient with alcohol or substance use disorder at every clinical encounter.

Detoxification

Patients should be motivated and be helped to appreciate the disadvantages of substance abuse. So the aim of treatment is to put the patient off the substance without the patient developing withdrawal symptoms (detoxification). It is advisable to carry out detoxification in the hospital because of the dangers of serious withdrawal symptoms.

This is achieved by:

- Giving a patient a drug that has the same properties as the drug of abuse (analogue) and then slowly reducing the dosage.
- In the case of alcohol the drug (analogue) used is Librium (Chlordiazepoxide), given 25 mg three times a day and gradually reducing the dosage over a period of 3-6 weeks.
- In addition, the individual with alcohol use disorder may be given an anticonvulsant such as Phenytoin 50 mg twice daily, or carbamazepine 200-400 mg twice daily for 2 weeks to guard against convulsions in a person who has history of seizures as a result of withdrawal symptoms. Vitamin B-Complex, 2 milliliters by the intra-muscular route daily to correct the associated lack of Vitamin B-group is given followed after 4-5 days by oral route.
- For other drugs, refer for appropriate management in the standard texts.
- Monitor the patient closely and correct any signs of circulatory failure by the use of intra-venous fluid therapy in the hospitalised patient.
- Rehabilitation: The patient is helped to rediscover his/her lost social and occupational skills.
- Support groups: Encourage formation and use of support groups such as alcoholic anonymous groups.

16
Mental Health Aspects of HIV/AIDS

EMILIO OVUGA

Introduction

AIDS is a late-stage manifestation of HIV infection, which is a chronic disease that runs its course over many years ending in death. With the availability of drugs to treat HIV/AIDS most persons infected with HIV will live longer with the infection and its associated psychosocial problems.

HIV/AIDS will perhaps remain the world's most dreaded epidemic of all time. A diagnosis of the condition puts a rude end to personal plans and effectively confronts the individual with the reality of an unexpected death (Ovuga, 1997). In the words of one individual with HIV/AIDS co morbid with Kaposi sarcoma, "A diagnosis of AIDS is like receiving death sentence in a court of law; a one way ticket to death". Being able to provide help to persons living with HIV/AIDS requires an understanding of the personal and social impacts of the condition on the lives of affected persons and their significant social relations.

Origins of mental health problems in HIV/AIDS

The psychiatric manifestations of HIV/AIDS are multiple and these may be due to the following:

- The virus invades the brain in up to 90% of cases. Viral invasion of the brain results in acute inflammation, micro-abscesses, vacuolation, and other degenerative changes.
- When an infected person moves from non-clinical to clinical AIDS stage; from being asymptomatic to being sick with symptoms of infection.
- Suspicion that one may be HIV-positive.
- Physical changes associated with disease, e.g. progressive weight loss, skin rashes, and loss of functional ability to carry out daily activities.

- Opportunistic infections, e.g. tuberculosis, cryptococcal infection, toxoplasmosis.
- Secondary spread of cancer, e.g. lymphoma, kaposi sarcoma.
- News of positive HIV-test result.

Psychosocial impact of HIV/AIDS

The reactions of the individual with HIV/AIDS comprise of worrying over his/her sexual conduct, the conduct of sexual partners, his/her plans for personal advancement, his/her failure to live up to the expectations of family friends and relatives, the prospect of passing through the long and painful process of dying and eventual death, and the misfortune of having to be the one to be infected. The affected person may experience episodes of panic attack with loss of sleep, appetite, and loss of interest in usual daily activities related to the fear of impending suffering, death and the reactions of family and friends. The person may be resentful and the provision of social care may be hampered by unpredictable outbursts of irritability and anger directed at those who provide nursing care either at home or at health facility. In later stages the individual may experience powerlessness, helplessness, sense of aloneness, and lack of self-worth, or the urgent need to accomplish unfinished business before dying. Suicidal thoughts leading to suicide or suicide attempt may occur.

While wealthy individuals with HIV/AIDS may not experience serious economic consequences, poor patients and their families will experience the problems of nutrition, and inability to meet medical costs of treatment thus hastening disease progression. Children of school age may drop out of school. Stigmatization and discrimination may make employment impossible, or lead to loss of employment. Chronic physical weakness may seriously interfere with activities of daily living. Physical pain or emotional distress may lead to the development of alcohol dependence. Psychiatric disorder may arise in individuals with prior history of mental illness and or substance dependence, and or those with family history of mental disorder.

Clinical aspects of HIV disease

The signs and symptoms of HIV/AIDS are so common that even non-health professionals can make spot diagnosis of the condition. The following list provides a quick review of the diverse clinical picture that patients with mental disorder due to HIV/AIDS might present with.

- Head, eyes, ears, nose and throat, e.g. oral thrush, oral ulcerations, silky hair, alopecia, gingivitis, stomatitis, etc.
- Respiratory tract, e.g. pulmonary tuberculosis, pneumonia.
- Gastrointestinal tract involvement, e.g. diarrhea, ulcers.
- Hematologic, e.g. anemia, neutropenia, thrombocytopenia.
- Dermatologic, e.g. skin rashes, herpes zoster rash, Kaposi sarcoma, etc.
- Central nervous system disease, e.g. seizure disorder, motor abnormality
- Effect of medication, e.g. alopecia, diarrhea, etc.
- Susceptibility to infections

Neurocognitive disorders

Evidence of disorder in cognitive functioning may occur both in HIV-infected individuals who are asymptomatic as well as those with active symptoms of AIDS disease. Features of cognitive dysfunction among asymptomatic individuals include:

- Impaired attention and concentration
- Psychomotor slowing, clumsiness
- Mild memory impairment leading to absent-mindedness, misplacing items, forgetfulness
- Difficulty with abstract thinking, divided attention, shifting cognitive sets, etc.

Features of cognitive impairment in symptomatic individuals include:

- Problems with language
- Visual and spatial disorientation
- Apraxias
- Movement disorders
- Behavioural disorders

Psychiatric disorders in HIV/AIDS

Moderate to severe psychiatric illness is prevalent among people with HIV/AIDS in health facilities in the order of 70-85%, and should always be searched for in persons attending HIV/AIDS clinic. Psychiatric disorders respond positively to treatment making it possible for the quality of life of the affected person to improve significantly. With the availability of effective antiretroviral medication, the prognosis of psychiatric illness in HIV disease is good, and most individuals could be weaned off psychotropic medication after the control of psychiatric symptoms. Psychiatric illness is also important for the additional reason that it may increase the risk of further HIV re-infection and or spread if left untreated. Thus the recognition and treatment of psychiatric illness as well as the underlying HIV/AIDS is necessary.

The recognition diagnosis and management of psychiatric disorders follows the same principles as appear in any textbook of mental health. It is important to remember that these disorders might arise in individuals who may otherwise show no outward signs and symptoms of HIV infection. It is therefore important that HIV infection should be suspected in an individual with a sudden onset of psychiatric illness.

- Adjustment disorder with depressed or anxious mood
- Manic disorder
- Depressive disorder
- Anxiety disorders, (panic disorder, Generalised anxiety disorder, obsessive-compulsive disorder), and agoraphobia (fear of open spaces)
- Schizophrenia-like illness
- HIV-associated dementia
- Delirium
- Alcohol or other substance dependence
- Suicide and attempted suicide

Clinical assessment

HIV/AIDS is a disease that involves all body systems and affects virtually all spheres of the life of the individual. Manifestations of the disease may depend on the clinical stage of the illness, ranging from cognitive dysfunction in the asymptomatic individual to the psychotic person. The following areas should be covered in the assessment as in any psychiatric history.

- Demographic data
- Presenting problems

- Psychiatric history
- Personal history, including educational background, employment history
- Social history, including family and marital histories
- Medical history
- Alcohol or other drug use history
- Sexual history, risk level, number of sexual partners
- Social support system
- Individual coping skills
- Personal strengths
- Financial and other resources
- Religious affiliation and spiritual practices
- Mental status assessment
- Evaluation of physical status
- Overall clinical assessment of the problem

Management objectives

As the individual living with HIV/AIDS faces multiple challenges and obstacles, clinical management should cover all possible aspects of his/her difficulty and should aim to achieve:

- Rapid and early control of distressing symptoms
- Limit progression of clinical status, e.g. neurocognitive decline
- Prevent or limit relapse into active psychiatric illness
- Improve quality of living
- Enhance return to employment as it applies
- Promote independent living as it applies
- Mobilise social support system
- Link the patient to appropriate sources of social resources
- Help individual adjust to his/her situation for positive living

Management principles

1. Enhance access to affordable or free transportation to attend clinical review, assistance to obtain food, clothing, provide child care, help with house work and general cleaning, and access new stock of medication.
2. The possible range of services include psychotherapy, rehabilitation services, other social support services, clinical care and planning for the future. Care plans should be adapted to meet the changing clinical needs of every patient over time.
3. Clinical and service providers involving several disciplines might wish to use the team approach to service and care provision to meet each patient's needs.
4. Service plans should be sensitive to the individuals' social background and take into account their cultural expectations as far as is possible.
5. Clinical outcome will be optimised when care providers relate to patients with respect that promotes the self-worth and dignity of the patients.
6. Clinical care should promote healthier behaviour and the need to reduce risky behaviour should be one of the primary goals of therapy.
7. Empower patients and their social support systems to be responsible for making important decisions regarding their care.

Management activities and guidelines

The following activities should form part of the overall services that should be considered for the individual living with HIV/AIDS.

- Assess clinical status to determine the nature of current mental health disorder, associated underlying and aggravating factors and potential protective factors.
- Assess the patient's individual needs for comprehensive care and management.

- Develop a service plan that incorporates all issues identified during assessment.
- Link the patient to available services.
- Monitor the patient's progress as the patient's needs are likely to be dynamic and change from time to time. It is important that attention is paid to potential side-effects of psychotropic medication, side-effects of antiretroviral medication and adverse reactions arising from drug-drug interaction.
- Carry out activities to prevent relapse, promote mental health, promote positive living and reduce risky behaviour.
- Involve the patient and or significant care provider in his social support system.

Psychotherapy

Individual psychotherapy

One-to-one psychotherapy or Counselling to address patient concerns regarding his/her HIV status as well as clinical management.

Group psychotherapy

Psychotherapy conducted for groups of patients facilitate change and manage mental health issues in HIV/AIDS among individual group members. In group psychotherapy individual members derive inspiration from the experience of other members and take responsibility for personal decisions and managing their mental health and HIV/AIDS issues. Group psychotherapy sessions may be facilitated by a team member or a professional.

Psychoeducation

Psychoeducation is a form of psychotherapy whose goal is to provide information on HIV/AIDS to patients and their care-givers. This form of psychotherapy may be provided by the clinician or invited guest speakers to groups of patients, and may cover topics such as safe sex, discordant couples, medication and its side-effects, HIV/AIDS in pregnancy and during lactation, managing mental health problems, etc.

Couple and family therapy
This form of psychotherapy provides opportunity for the spouse and or significant other family members to join and stay in therapy to optimize the positive outcome of psychosocial interventions. Through family therapy, dysfunctional family relationships may be addressed to promote adequate clinical improvement.

Cognitive behavioural therapy
Cognitive behavioural therapy addresses negative irrational belief systems and accompanying dysfunctional behavioural practices of individuals.

Themes in psychotherapy for HIV/AIDS

Individual patients may experience or bring several issues to psychotherapy sessions.

Self-esteem
The vulnerable individual with HIV/AIDS may experience loss of self-esteem, shame, guilt and self-blame for having been infected by HIV. These experiences may contribute to depression and suicidal behaviour.

Parenting
The demands associated with HIV/AIDS may disrupt normal parenting and this may further aggravate the already low self-esteem of vulnerable parent.

Fear
People living with HIV/AIDS may experience excessive fear regarding rejection and loss of social support, disease progression and impact on their lives, and the pain of death and dying, etc, and may seem to demand too much from their care providers at home or in hospital.

Disclosure
As a result of fear the person living with HIV/AIDS may choose not to disclose his/her HIV-status and risk infecting the possibly HIV-negative spouse and or risk giving birth to an infected newborn.

Loss of loved ones

Prior bereavement(s) as a result of HIV/AIDS may aggravate the psychological trauma of a person who contracts HIV. Survivor guilt may be evident and the older individual living with HIV may wish to die and join lost family members.

Issue of compliance

Compliance may be affected by the mental status of the individual, duration of illness, the availability and cost of medication, and the degree of adaptation of the individual to ill health.

Lazarus syndrome

As an individual with a long history of illness with HIV notices significant improvement, he/she may experience significant level of increased energy, well-being and a significant reduction of symptoms. Conversely an individual may paradoxically experience symptoms of depression, sadness, social isolation and impairment in social functioning. This latter reaction may be associated with severe depression and suicidal behaviour, which may interfere with compliance leading to premature death.

Religious belief

People who live with HIV often develop strong religious and spiritual beliefs that help them cope with their situation, stimulate personal resources for living and integrate meaning into their experience of living with HIV. Other individuals may reject medication or any other form of intervention if they believe that they have been "cured by Christ". It is therefore important to evaluate the religious and spiritual belief systems of the patient living with HIV and to help them accept the reality of AIDS without ARVs.

Barriers to mental health care

People living with HIV/AIDS face several barriers to access to mental health services. These barriers are grouped into the following categories.

a) Barriers related to personal factors

(i) Negative personal reaction to the diagnosis of HIV/AIDS may hinder seeking help

(ii) Concomitant presence of mental disorder may lead to impaired ability to seek health care.

(iii) Multiple clinical problems might make it difficult for patients to cope with the demands of multiple drug therapy and regimes. Further more drug-drug interactions might interfere with access to mental health care.

(iv) Economic impoverishment may prevent the patient from accessing mental health services if services are not free.

(v) A socially isolated patient may fail to access and or sustain mental health services in the long-term.

b) Barriers related to the health care system

(i) Fragmentation of the health care system may hinder access to care for mental health problems

(ii) Lack of knowledge and skills among health care providers may make it harder for mental health problems to be recognised, diagnosed and treated.

c) Barriers related to societal attitudes practices and prejudice

(i) Negative attitudes among health care providers may hinder their ability to provide appropriate care to persons living with HIV/AIDS.

(ii) Societal and cultural beliefs and practices that view HIV/AIDS as being due to witchcraft or due to the actions of supernatural powers may prevent patients from accessing appropriate mental health services early.

Integration of HIV/AIDS services

To be effective, services for individuals who suffer from mental illness and are also HIV-positive should be integrated into general health and social sector services that range from providing legal service in drafting a will or other legal document; helping family members access basic human needs such as food, shelter, clothing; helping children obtain education; and referring the patient to other medical specialists for appropriate services.

17
Mental Health Aspects of Obstetrics and Gynaecology

JULIET NAKKU

Post-natal mental disorders

Postnatal mental disorders are a group of psychiatric illnesses, which affect up to 15% of women during the first 4 weeks following childbirth. The disorders most commonly affect women who have had their first child and may interfere with the mother's ability to establish emotional attachment with their newborn, communicate with the baby and provide overall maternal care to the newborn. Although postnatal mental disorders are common, they are rarely recognised and correctly treated.

Women at risk of getting psychiatric symptoms in pregnancy

These are women:

- With the story of previous mental illness in the individual and the family
- With serious medical problems affecting the course of pregnancy, e.g. diabetes.
- Who need social support and care.
- With alcohol and or substance abuse problems.
- Who are on psychiatric medication, e.g. Lithium; the women risk getting babies with malformation, impaired growth and prenatal problems.

Other Conditions that predispose women to psychiatric problems related to childbirth include:

- Hyperemesis Gravidarum
- Nausea and vomiting in the first these of pregnancy
- Pseudocyesis women who believe they are pregnant while they are not
- Couvade syndrome - husband believes he is experiencing symptom of being pregnant.

- Unwanted pregnancy resulting into termination of pregnancy due to psychological cause
- Women with spontaneous abortion.
- Women with therapeutic abortion.

Types of postnatal mental disorder

There are three types of postnatal mental disorder:

- Maternity blues
- Postnatal depression
- Post-partum psychosis.

Maternity blues

Maternity blues are a group of symptoms that occur within 3-4 days following childbirth and comprise of sadness, tearfulness, poor sleep, poor appetite, irritable mood, and symptoms of anxiety. Symptoms of maternity blues occur among 50% of women after childbirth, are self-limiting in the majority of cases, and remit on reassurance of the mother concerned, and rarely last 1-2 weeks. No definitive treatment is required in most cases.

Maternity blues are common and may resolve on reassurance only. However, adequate assessment is required to ensure that mothers with depression and eventual severe mental illness receive effective and appropriate treatment early.

Postnatal depression

Postnatal depression affects 10-20% of first-time mothers and begins 2-4 weeks after childbirth, usually after discharge from hospital. Postnatal depression can be recognised by routine inquiry for the symptoms of depression during the times the mother attends well-baby clinics, particularly during the first 4 weeks after childbirth. In the absence of direct inquiry for it, postnatal depression may become chronic and may interfere with the mother's ability to take care of the newborn adequately. The symptoms of postnatal depression include:

- Depressed sad mood
- Loss of interest in usual activities, including interest in the baby
- Reduced or disturbed sleep
- Disturbed or loss of appetite for food

- Loss or increased weight
- Loss of energy
- Feelings of guilt
- Poor concentration
- Ideas of inadequacy and worthlessness
- Suicidal wishes or death wishes

Postnatal depression is best managed through early identification by careful history aimed to detect postnatal depression in a mother with a baby of less than twelve weeks old and who has come to attend postnatal clinic for herself or for the welfare of the newborn. Following a positive identification, the mother should be helped to share her feelings regarding her status and role as mother, her feelings toward the newborn, and the quality of social support system available to her. If the woman has suicidal thoughts in addition to other symptoms of depression, medication with an antidepressant is recommended.

Post-partum psychosis

Post-partum mental disorder is common, affecting 10-20% of mothers within 2-12 weeks after childbirth. Post-partum mental illness can be detected early on the basis of the mother's physical health, history of mental illness and the level of social support available to her.

However, this disorder affects less than 1% of women after childbirth. It usually begins within the first two weeks of childbirth and is so severe that it may threaten the normal mother-child relationship, the security of the newborn and is associated with a high risk of suicide or infanticide.

Postpartum psychosis is characterised by agitation, hallucinations and delusions similar to other acute and severe mental illness in the category of psychosis such as schizophrenia, mania. The affected mother may hold bizarre and prominent delusions about herself and or her baby including the belief that the newborn is a monster, deformed, not a human or a dangerous creature.

Post-partum psychosis may take the form of delirium, mania or schizophrenic disorder.

Confirmation of the diagnosis may be made when the following points are present.

Mental

- Sudden onset, varying symptoms of psychosis may present
- Suicidal tendencies
- Infanticide
- Loss of affection to baby and husband.

Physical

- History of recent childbirth
- Poor hygiene
- Constipation may be present especially in depression
- Headache, dry furred tongue
- Increased pulse rate associated with puerperal sepsis.
- Breast engorgement due to sudden withdrawal of breast feeding

Risk factors for post-partum psychosis

- First child
- Previous major psychiatric illness affecting the woman
- Family history of mental illness
- Inadequate social support, particularly from the spouse
- Early separation from mother
- Infection within the first two to four weeks following childbirth

Post-partum psychosis is managed through:

- History taking, physical examination, mental status assessment and appropriate laboratory investigations to exclude an underlying physical condition that might be responsible for the episode of mental disorder.
- Admission to hospital for adequate control of illness symptoms, closer observation, and optima investigations. Admission of the baby may be considered if there is no risk of hospital infection, if there is no one to care for the baby at home, and if the mother is not outright rejecting the baby. Admission of the baby with the mother is expected to preserve the mother-child relationship and ensures that the mother continues to breastfeed the baby.

- Medication depends on the predominant nature of symptom groups, such as depression, mania, schizophrenia or delirium.

Prevention of post-partum mental disorder

- Proper and adequate screening of mothers at ante-natal and post-natal clinic aimed to detect and treat early cases of mental disorder
- Treatment of any post-partum infection
- Counseling for maternity blues and post-natal depression
- Encouraging mothers with a history of psychiatric illness to remain in contact with their doctors

Management of an episode of post-partum mental disorder

The management of post-partum mental disorder is similar to that of any other psychiatric disorder. For a detailed guide of management the health worker is referred to the relevant description of the major types of psychiatric disorder. The more likely disorders that one might manage include one of the following:

- Affective disorder (manic or depressive phase)
- Schizophrenia
- Other forms of unspecified psychosis
- Delirium (usually due to infection and or poor nutritional status

A decision has, however, to be made early in the course of care planning as to whether the affected mother should be admitted to hospital or could be better managed under the care of family at home. If admission is required a decision should also be made as to whether she should be admitted along with the infant or not. Normally admission will be recommended if:

- the illness episode is severe and cannot be managed at home and or requires biomedical investigations that cannot be carried out if the woman is not in hospital
- management requires supervision
- there is insufficient social support at home

It would be advisable to have the mother admitted with her baby unless there are specific contra-indications to the admission of the baby. Admission is beneficial as it enhances the early development of mother-infant bondage and prevents the drying up of the mother's breast milk. If admission is possible it is further recommended that a relative stays around to support the mother with breast-feeding and in the provision of general welfare needs to the baby and mother. Special care should be taken to ensure that the infant does not get hospital infection while in the ward. In addition if evidence of possible infanticide is noticed extra care should be taken by hospital staff (in the case of the admitted mother) and family to ensure that the baby is protected from potential harm. It will be necessary to continue providing this protection till the time when the mother has developed insight into her mental state and has sufficient mental capacity to understand her relationship to her newborn baby.

18

Psychological Impact of Trauma

EMILIO OVUGA

Introduction

The psychological outcomes of the experience of trauma are so real that it may be difficult even for victims themselves to believe in them. Yet disasters, whether natural as in the form of a house collapsing or man-made as in the case of repeated domestic violence and genocide, are common place. This chapter outlines key issues about the psychological consequences of trauma also known as Post-traumatic Stress Disorder (PTSD).

Definition

PTSD is mental disorder that follows the experience of severe trauma that is beyond the tolerance of the ordinary human being.

Prevalence

The exact figure of how common PTSD is remains difficult to say. What is clear is that soon after the occurrence of trauma affecting whole communities the prevalence of symptoms of PTSD can be detected among 80-90%. However, as time elapses, this prevalence will drop considerably over the next six months to about a third of the population, and this figure will continue to drop over the next year or so to less than 10%.

Causes

The causes of PTSD may be categorized into two broad groups as depicted in Table 18.1 below.

Table 18.1: Causes of post-traumatic stress disorder

Natural disaster	Man made disaster
Storm	Domestic violence
Floods	Rape and defilement
Bush fire	Armed conflict

Natural disaster	Man made disaster
Earthquake	War
Bus or other accident	Political terror
	Suicide bombing
	Hostage taking

The causes of PTSD vary as is shown in the summary in table 1 and they range from rape, child abuse, and domestic violence to armed conflict and war, suicide bombing or political terror meted out on the populace by their own governments as an instrument of domination (Herman, 1992). The common factor in these varied causes of trauma is the intense feeling of danger, the imminent threat of death and personal annihilation, the loss of control, and the intense feeling of helplessness.

Trauma may be experienced directly by the victim, perpetrator, rescue team members and media personnel or indirectly by other people through witnessing when one is present at the time of the occurrence of the trauma, report made by witnesses, viewing the events of the trauma on television, reading about the trauma or seeing the photographs of trauma events and victims.

Who is liable to suffer from PTSD?

PTSD may affect literally every one who is exposed to the events leading to trauma. Those affected may include both the perpetrator of the trauma and the victim directly or indirectly as well as bystanders or other people who witness, are informed, who view or read about the events of trauma in the print or electronic media.

Painful experiences of trauma

People who are trapped in trauma situations experience

- ***Terror*** – intense fear that eventually fades away to leave the victim feeling helpless
- ***Disconnection*** – the individual feels cut-off, separated from family and friends; he/she becomes isolated
- ***Captivity*** – the individual feels trapped, prisoner, in the full control of the trauma situation; he/she depends on the trauma situation or on fate for his/her personal safety and survival

- ***Sense of abandonment; loss of trust*** – in the hour of need the individual lacks access to sources of any help and support

Issues in trauma experience

Though the painful occurrence of trauma is common, society and individual members of the society often advocate for victims to remain silent, adhere to the unspoken oath of secrecy and to deny the reality of the trauma at all costs. This is expected as to admit the experience of trauma may be seen a sign of moral weakness, and may attract guilt feelings and self-blame for exposing oneself to the events of trauma; society often blames victims for their part in the events of trauma.

Manifestations of trauma experience

Many victims learn to cope with their trauma experiences in the community partly with support from their communities and partly learning to live with the aftermath of trauma experience. Those individuals who fail to cope with symptoms of PTSD may use alcohol excessively for self-medication against anxiety, depression and early severe mental illness and to induce sleep, or engage in suicide behaviour. Children cope with their trauma experience by replaying the events of trauma that they might have witnessed or experienced. For example it has been common for children from northern Uganda to re-enact the horrifying events of raids by the Lord's Resistance Army during play times.

Symptoms and signs of PTSD

- Disbelief; unwillingness to accept that the events of trauma have occurred
- Emotional numbness; being unable to feel sad or joyful
- Impaired capacity for human relations; being unable to form warm trusting relations with other persons, particularly members of the opposite sex as occurs after rape
- Sleep disturbance; poor or total lack of sleep due to frightening dreams about the events of trauma
- Loss of appetite for food
- Flashbacks; experiencing the events of trauma in full wakefulness, e.g. hearing victims crying and pleading for mercy like a flash of lightning

- Hallucinations; experiencing the events of trauma in great detail in full wakefulness, e.g. the act of torturing and killing a victim
- Re-experience of trauma in situations that serve as reminders of trauma, e.g. every time people who have been abducted by the Lord's Resistance Army pass by where they were abducted from they re-experience the full events of the abduction
- Avoidance of situations that remind the victim of the trauma
- Irritability; getting upset easily
- Unpredictable reactions of aggression and violence
- Increased fear reaction; being jumpy at every sound, being ready to flee
- Depression, anxiety, alcohol abuse, suicidal behaviour
- More complicated signs:
    - Contradictory behaviour, as if there are more individuals in one body
    - An individual's behaviour changes unpredictably from warm friendly to being upset or violent
    - An individual loses function of part of the body, e.g. being blind, deaf or paralysed when he/she is not
    - Having numerous symptoms, such as body pains and aches that do not respond to medication

Complications of PTSD

Common complications in PTSD include:

- Alcohol abuse
- Suicidal behaviour
- Chronic depression
- Anxiety disorder

Helping people with trauma

Helping people with trauma in primary care requires that one recognises them in the first place, and this may not be easy. A useful tip to remember is that the next person at the clinic may be one with the problems of trauma; Uganda is a traumatised society and people with trauma may be common in primary care.

Useful clues to the recognition of individuals with the effects of trauma are:

- Multiple body pains and aches
- Problem of alcohol or other drug abuse
- Vague general symptoms
- Individual comes from current or previous war zone
- Individual is a child or young adult of both sexes

The psychological approach to helping is perhaps the best approach to care as this method will help the individual achieve reconnection to other caring human beings, regain lost control and autonomy, regain lost trust and confidence, achieve a validation of his/her experiences and escape from captivity through talk therapy. To help the individual achieve these objectives the following five questions in talk therapy may be asked over a course of 4 to 6 sessions:

1. How has the experience of trauma affected your life personally? (e.g. change in the person of the individual, behaviour patterns, feelings, thoughts)
2. What are the main problems that you have experienced often or repeatedly as a result of the trauma? (e.g. occupation, human relations)
3. How have you coped with the problems that you have mentioned or talked about? (E.g. what has he/she done about personal experiences? Does he/she use prayers, isolate self, use alcohol, or feel suicidal?)
4. How else could you deal with these problems? (E.g. what alternative ways are available for getting over the effects of the trauma? who are there to confide in?)
5. How do you plan to reconstruct your life from now on? (e.g. What plans are available for the future, to get over the trauma and move on?)

Appropriate medication to treat depression, anxiety or other form of mental disorder may be used if indicated. Very often the need for medication will disappear as the individual improves on talk therapy. When in doubt refer to a senior early.

19

Dementia

EMILIO OVUGA

Definition

Dementia is a mental disorder of gradual onset and with a progressive down hill course. It is characterised by multiple intellectual deficits which include:

- Memory impairment and one or more of the following:
- Difficulty in speech (aphasia).
- Difficulty in carrying out motor activities (apraxia).
- Difficulty in recognising familiar objects including family members (agnosia).
- Difficulty in carrying out complex intellectual functions such as planning, sequencing, organising, implementing, abstract thinking, and evaluating.

Prevalence

The prevalence of dementia in Uganda is unknown but individuals with this condition do present themselves to the primary care clinician. The one-year prevalence of dementia has been estimated elsewhere at 2-4% of adults aged 65 years and 20% for those aged 85 years (APA, 1992).

Classification of dementia

There are two types of dementia. Dementia beginning after the age of 65 years is known as senile dementia or more accurately, Alzheimer's dementia. Dementia that occurs in adults of younger age is known as pre-senile dementia.

Causes of dementia

1. The cause of Alzheimer's dementia is associated with genetic predisposition that leads to the accumulation of harmful chemical substances in the brain.

2. The cause of pre-senile dementia is usually an acquired injury to the brain, such as severe brain injury in a motor vehicle accident, infections such as HIV, meningitis; brain tumour; or from the below optimal functioning of the thyroid gland. In addition:
   a) Severe depression in adults below the age of 65 may present with features of dementia, which is known as depressive pseudo-dementia.
   b) Deficiencies of vitamins B1, B2 have been associated with pellagra associated with dermatitis (skin rashes on the exposed parts of the body, stomatitis with beefy red tongue); diarrhoea; and dementia (confusion and memory failure).

Examples of clinical symptoms and signs

Memory

The individual may be unable to learn any new information and will fail to remember facts; he/she may keep a diary of planned activities so as not to forget; may go to the shop or market to purchase items and may fail to buy any as a result of having forgotten the items.

Disorientation

The individual may get lost even within his/her place of residence. The person may walk out of the home and fail to trace his/her way back till family and friends bring him/her back. Confusion due to disorientation may lead to lack of sleep and restlessness at night, predisposing the person to injuries.

Impaired intellectual functioning

During the early stages of the illness the individual may complain of difficulty in concentrating at work, of being unable to perform his/her usual duties that require thinking, or of getting easily tired.

Motor functioning

In late stages the individual with dementia may fail to carry out even simple motor activities, such as walking or sitting.

Social dysfunction

Confusion may lead to lack of sleep, restlessness, and agitation at night, the patient getting lost, and the family experiencing extra strain in having to manage the patient. These problems may predispose the patient to injury of self or other family members.

Management

- Take detailed history followed by comprehensive physical and mental status examination.
- Carry out appropriate biomedical investigations indicated by findings on history and physical examination, e.g.

- Haemogram - haemoglobin, erythrocyte sedimentation rate, red blood count, total and differential white cell count, film comment, packed cell volume, mean corpuscular haemoglobin.
- Urine analysis - sugar, proteins, casts, cells, relevant culture studies as indicated
- Renal function tests
- Liver function tests
- CSF studies
- VDRL, TPHA
- Thyroid function tests
- ECG; EEG; Skull x-rays; CT scan.

- The family should keep the patient's environment simple and relatively structured.
- Ensure adequate nutrition and fluid intake
- Teach the patient simple measures of personal care and hygiene as necessary.

- Draw the attention of the family to the memory impairment that the patient suffers from. The family should be tolerant to the patient's behavioural problems and constantly remind the patient of what to do or what happened a few minutes or hours ago, but in a gentle uncritical manner.
- Respect and protect the dignity and autonomy of the individual concerned.

Drugs

Several drugs have been developed but many are not available in Uganda due to high costs. A combination of high-potency vitamins containing vitamins B_1, B_2, C, E that are available on the open market in Uganda are reported to improve intellectual functioning of the brain in dementia. In general treatment in dementia may be limited to symptomatic control, such as the control of hallucinations, delusions, symptoms of co-existing depression, or symptoms of infection.

20
Epilepsy

EMILIO OVUGA

Introduction

Epilepsy is the commonest neurological disorder in Uganda. The diagnosis of epilepsy is often not readily accepted, particularly by the carer of the patient with the condition. The disorder presents in several different ways and this complicates attempts at diagnosis. It is however important that the correct diagnosis of epilepsy is made early to prevent neurological complications, promote adequate control and improve the welfare and quality of life of those affected.

Epidemiology

The prevalence of epilepsy in Uganda ranges from 0.21% to 2% (Ovuga et al, 1992). Health facility records in Uganda indicate that epilepsy is one of the commonest health problems affecting the nervous system while globally epilepsy is estimated to affect 0.5% of the population. In Uganda epilepsy is commonest among communities affected by river blindness disease that affects the whole of the western part of Uganda from Kisoro to north western Uganda. Though the role of consumption of poorly cooked pork in causing epilepsy in Uganda has not been evaluated, eating poorly prepared pork has been documented to be the major cause of epilepsy in Eastern, Central and Southern Africa. Every effort should be made to define the importance of possible infection with pig tape worm as a cause of the individual case; epilepsy due to pig tape worm infection is highly curable and can be prevented through collaboration with veterinarians, agriculturalists, and communities through public health education and improved methods of pig production.

Aetiology

Epilepsy is a recurrent disorder characterised by outbursts of excessive activity in part or the whole brain, which occurs suddenly, disappears spontaneously and has a tendency to reoccur. It is also characterised by episodes of fits (attacks) of loss of consciousness with violent body movements. It is caused by abnormal electrical activity in the brain.

The commonest risk factor for epilepsy in Uganda is the experience of convulsions due to fever in early childhood at the age of 2-4 years. Forty percent of epilepsy sufferers give a positive history of such convulsions in early childhood and 35% of children who suffer from convulsions associated with fever have a positive family history of such convulsions. In other parts of Africa (e.g. Tanzania, Burundi, Mozambique, Zambia, Zimbabwe, South Africa, Cameroun, and Ghana), the rate of epilepsy has been found to be highest in communities with high concentrations of pig rearing and consumption.

Trigger Factors

Episodes of convulsions may be precipitated by a variety of physiological states including:

- Fever in childhood
- Sleep and convulsions during sleep may occur soon after the child has retired to bed or anytime from 1.00 am to 7.00 am in the morning
- Daylong or overnight fast
- Emotional arousal, e.g., fear, anger, excitement
- Flickering lights.
- Intoxication with or withdrawal from alcohol
- Fatigue and boredom

Classification of epilepsy:

Several types of epilepsy exist. However, the more common types in primary care are outlined below.

1. **Grand mal fits (Generalised tonic-clonic):** This is a sudden attack with loss of consciousness and violent body jerking lasting 3-5 minutes. The patient regains consciousness spontaneously and may sustain injuries during the episode, e.g. tongue biting or may become incontinent. Some times the patient may go into a confusional state and become aggressive. There are chances of having repeated fits. This is the commonest type of epilepsy in Uganda.

2. **Petit mal fits (absences):** There is temporary loss of consciousness and the patient, usually a child, has short disruption in motor activity, e.g. if a person was writing, he stops and the pen drops down. However, this type is difficult to recognise. The attacks may occur several times in a day and may present with poor academic performance in a school child; a child seeming to be careless or naughty and being prone to corporal punishment.

3. **Focal epilepsy (Jacksonian):** This type of epilepsy disrupts the function of a particular part of the body resulting from excessive electrical discharges from a focal point in the brain, which controls that part. For example if the focus of the epilepsy is the part of brain which supplies the left hand, there will be jerking of fingers and or the whole of that hand. The seizure may spread throughout the body and become a generalised.

4. **Temporal Lobe:** This is one of the commonest types of focal epilepsy. In this case the abnormal electrical discharge originates from temporal lobe of the brain. There is loss of memory, mood changes, and purposive or automatic purposeless behaviour with repetitive movements, such as chewing and swallowing movements or smacking of the lips, etc. There may be olfactory and auditory hallucinations. Outbursts of aggression is a common feature.

5. **Continuous fits (status epileptics):** This is a complication of grand mal epilepsy where fits follow one another without the patient regaining consciousness in between the fits. It is a dangerous condition, which should be treated as an emergency (see Psychiatric Emergencies).

Causes of grand mal epilepsy

In a majority of cases the cause is unclear but a number of factors may contribute to this condition. These include the following:

1. Heredity: There is a positive family history of epilepsy and the condition runs in the family

2. Uncontrolled convulsions in fever during the first 4 years of life (febrile convulsions)

3. Head injuries e.g. from accidents, domestic violence etc.

4. Birth trauma (injury) to an infant
5. Brain tumor (e.g. blood clot, brain abscess, benign or malignant growth)
6. Infections e.g. meningitis, HIV, encephalitis
7. Alcohol and drug abuse.

Signs and symptoms of grand mal epilepsy: -

- Sudden loss of consciousness followed by falling
- Stiffness of the whole body
- Jerking movements of the whole body
- There may be frothing at the mouth
- There may be tongue biting
- The patient may pass urine, feces or both
- After a fit some may fall into a deep sleep, others may not fall to sleep but appear confused for sometime and may wander off aimlessly.

Diagnosis

The diagnosis of epilepsy is clinical based on careful history taking. Some forms of epilepsy do not present with convulsions (see "different faces of epilepsy" below) and a high index of suspicion is required to enable appropriate history to be conducted. Investigative tools may be used in aiding the diagnosis of epilepsy, and these include:

- **Electroencephalography (EEG)** may reveal epileptiform activity. However, 20% of individuals with epilepsy have normal EEG, and 20% of people without epilepsy have abnormal EEG. In general, one in every two requests for EEG draws normal EEG reports.
- **Skull X-rays** may indicate evidence of lesions such as calcifications or evidence of increased pressure within the cranium. About one in every three carefully considered requests for skull x-rays yield positive results.
- **CT scanning** of the brain may confirm the presence of a tumour within the cranium. Only about 3% of requests for CT scanning may be positive.

The most reliable tool in the diagnosis of epilepsy is careful history taking, and where possible, the witnessing of an episode of attack of epilepsy. In most cases the diagnosis of a major tonic-clonic seizure is easy. The features of epilepsy, whether tonic-clonic or other form, are usually similar:

- The attacks are episodic; that is, the attacks come and go.
- The person is usually unaware of what is taking place, and will not respond to sensory stimulation at the time.
- The person will lack memory for events during the episode.
- The person's behaviour is usually normal between episodes.

Different faces of epilepsy

Epilepsy may present in one of several ways thus making it difficult to recognise. Remember that the classification provided in this book has been over-simplified and there are more classes of epilepsy than have been provided. The different ways in which the condition may broadly present include:

- Tonic-clonic seizures.
- Sensory manifestations.
- Motor manifestations.
- Behavioural manifestations.
- Emotional manifestations.
- Psychological manifestations.
- Autonomic manifestations.
- Memory disorder - e.g. sense of familiarity or sense of unfamiliarity.

Seizures occurring without motor manifestations, also referred to as non-convulsive seizures, may take the form of behavioural, emotional, psychological and cognitive disorders. Psychosis akin to bipolar affective disorder is one the commonest forms in which non-convulsive seizures may present in Uganda, leading to unnecessary admission and subsequent stigmatisation of the sufferer. This form of seizure disorder is also important for its association with crime during the commission of which the individual may appear normal before an untrained eye. When in doubt refer early to senior colleague.

Differential diagnosis of epilepsy

Other disorders need to be distinguished from epilepsy and these include:

- Simple fainting attacks.
- Syncope.
- Migraine headache.
- Bronchial asthma.
- Psychogenic seizures, previously known as hysterical convulsions.

The common terminology used by patients is "The Attack". The health worker needs to learn how to differentiate the above differential conditions from epilepsy as they may all be described at the bedside as "The attack".

Principles of management

- Explain your clinical opinion in simple language.
- Explain the treatment plan and ensure that you have been understood.
- Explain the drug dosage schedule, and where possible, provide written notes.
- Explain expected drug side-effects.
- Explain the expected course and outcome of treatment.
- Highlight the role of possible trigger factors and how to control them for optimal treatment outcome.
- Provide encouraging information and how to maximise positive treatment outcome.
- Encourage the adoption of active lifestyle and positive attitude in life.

Purpose of medication

Several new anticonvulsant medications have been developed. However, none of these is available in Uganda. The choice of anticonvulsant therapy will therefore be limited to Phenytoin sodium, carbamazepine, sodium valproate, and Ethosuximide. The use of these medications should be guided by the following principles.

- The management of epilepsy should aim at the control and or prevention of seizures without impairing the patient's social functioning in daily life.

- Take comprehensive history concerning clinical presentation, aetiological factors, social circumstances general health history, previous medications, etc.
- Carry out appropriate biomedical, social and psychological investigations.
- Choose appropriate medication based on assessment results.
- Use one drug at a time. Combination medication will be indicated in only a few cases.
- Decide on appropriate dose and dosage schedule based on clinical profile including seizure frequency, trigger factors, age of the patient and the most likely type of seizure disorder.
- Monitor clinical progress weekly or fortnightly initially. Adjust drug dosage and frequency according to treatment outcome.
- Refer the patient to a colleague early if you are in doubt or if no clinical progress is noted over a six-week period.

Management of grand mal fit

Management of grand mal fit is divided into two parts viz;

- Emergency Management of grand mal fit and
- General Management

In Emergency Management the followings are done;

(i) Keep calm

(ii) Protect the patient from hurting himself by removing him from danger e.g. fire, water, sharp instruments or any of dangerous environments.

(iii) Protect the fitting person's head with something soft or your hands.

(iv) Loosen tight clothing

(v) After the fit (convulsion) position the patient in the semi prone position to help in the breathing and recovery.

(vi) Stay with the person until he has fully recovered.

(vii) After recovery, re-orientate the patient and if he wishes, allow him to continue with what he was doing

(viii) Reassure the patient because he/she may feel embarrassed

(xi) In case of injuries, wash the wounds with soap and water and cover with clean cloth.

(x) Assist the patient to tidy up

CAUTION! Do not:

1. Try to put anything in the patient's mouth during the fit.
2. Give him anything to eat drink during the fit
3. Try to stop the jerking movement

General management of grand mal epilepsy

1. The caretaker/patient should record the fit in a book
2. Encourage the person or caretaker to seek medical attention from the nearest health facility
3. Encourage a person with epilepsy to take drugs as advised by the medical personnel.
4. The person on treatment should continue until advised by a medical worker.
5. A person with epilepsy should be followed up regularly.
6. Encourage the person with epilepsy/caretaker to join epilepsy support groups in their area.
7. Discuss the patient's social and personal problems associated with the epilepsy to enhance his/her adaptation in the community of family, friends, etc.

Drug treatment

The drugs used in the treatment of epilepsy do not cure but they control fits. The drugs of choice for treating Grand mal Epilepsy are:

- Phenytoin (Epanutin) tablets in the strength of 100 – 200 mgs taken 100-900 mg per day in 1 - 3 divided doses
- Carbamazepine (tegretol) tablets in the strengths of 200 mg taken 100-1200 mg daily in 1 - 3 divided doses
- Sodium valproate in the strength of 200 mg taken 200-1200 mg per day in

Review clinical progress after every 2-4 weeks on out-patient basis till control is achieved, and every 2-3 days for in-patient till active seizures cease. The maximum dose for each patient depends on control of fits and tolerance of side effects.

Surgical treatment of epilepsy

Surgery for the treatment of epilepsy is reserved for cases that have failed to respond on adequate doses of the appropriate medication for a period of two years. In such cases seizures may involve the tip of the temporal lobe associated with severe scarring of the brain tissue; in other cases surgery may be indicated if there is demonstrable evidence of a tumor being the cause, such as tape worm cyst, and abscess or hematoma.

Surgical intervention is not without its own hazards such as permanent and irreversible personality change and decline in intellectual capacity, and should be considered only after all due investigations and consultations have been made including:

- Neuropsychological tests by the clinical psychologist to ascertain that the individual's personality and intelligence are adequate and will not decline to a level lower than that reasonable to support independent life.
- Neuro-imaging investigations to confirm the presence of a lesion that can be excised without cause undue injury to healthy brain tissue
- Detailed mental status assessment by the psychiatrist to assure that the surgery will not add further burden to that already imposed by surgery
- There should be ample evidence to show that appropriate investigations have been conducted and that the correct medication for two years have failed to bring about optimal control of seizures and improvement in the quality of life of the person affected supported by measurable clinical criteria
- The surgery should be considered after securing informed consent of either the patient who has sufficient mental capacity to understand explanations, or the relatives, or both
- In any case the decision to go ahead with surgery for epilepsy should be considered by a Board of Experts that includes the neurologist, neuro-psychiatrist, clinical psychologist, neuro-surgeon, the social worker and a legal advisor.

Treatment of continuous fits (status epilepticus)

Children:

- For children 10 years of age or less, give rectal Diazepam (Valium) 5 mg immediately and refer.

Adults:

- Rectal diazepam (valium) 20 mg immediately and refer.

Criteria for referral

1. Continuous fits
2. Patients less than 2 years of age
3. Patients who have fits in pregnancy only
1. Patients with fits occurring only in the presence of fever.
2. Failure to control fits if a patient gets more than 3 fits a day
3. Patients on phenobarbitone and are developing any of the following:
   - Vomiting for more than 48 hours
   - Skin rash
   - Yellow coloring of eyes
   - Reddening of the eyes
   - Hyperactivity.
   - Irritability
   - Sore throat

Education of caretakers and persons with epilepsy

All persons involved in the management of epilepsy should know that Epilepsy is not infectious but can be controlled on drugs.

- Personal risks: Some activities in a person's life may expose them to risks of injury due to the unpredictable nature and timing of fits. Persons with epilepsy should not engage in activities near large body of water alone, e.g. well, river while fetching water, swimming etc.
- Persons with epilepsy should be advised not to work at heights, e.g. Climbing or working at a height at construction site, electricity pole, etc.

- Individuals with epilepsy should be advised not to operate machines e.g. driving vehicles, riding, welding, etc. till when they have been seizure-free on medication for a period of 3 years.
- Patients with epilepsy should be advised to refrain from drinking alcohol as alcohol increases the risk of seizures.
- Epilepsy is not caused by witchcraft or evil spirits.
- Contact with feces, saliva, urine or flatus of a fitting person can not transmit the disorder of epilepsy.
- Epilepsy can be controlled with drugs taken regularly
- Persons with epilepsy are not "mad" and do not suffer from mental disorder; epilepsy falls within the specialty of neurologists and people with epilepsy should ideally be referred to neurologists.
- Children with epilepsy can benefit from schooling like any other children.
- Persons with epilepsy should participate in community activities along with other members of their communities.
- Sharing utensils (cups, plates, spoons etc) does not pass on the disease
- Flickering lights e.g. video halls, welding can precipitate epilepsy.

Outcomes in the management of epilepsy

Patient not improving satisfactorily

The optimal control of psychiatric symptoms on optimal doses of drugs is usually achieved after at least two weeks, and adequate improvement may not be noticed until after four weeks. If a patient is not improving satisfactorily, consider the following and take appropriate steps to improve clinical and psychosocial outcomes of care.

- Inadequate or excessive dosing may be responsible.
- Patient is probably not taking medication as instructed.
- Patient did not receive adequate instruction.
- The diagnosis may be wrong.
- Treatment may be wrong.
- A medical condition might be responsible for the mental symptoms but it has not been recognised for treatment

- Lack of improvement may be due to side-effects of medication.
- Multiple drug therapy may be responsible.
- Patient suffers from two or more conditions each requiring attention.
- Overall health and mental health status is poor and requires attention.

Febrile convulsions

Febrile convulsions are convulsive episodes that occur in response to a sudden rise of body temperature, usually above 39 degrees Celsius. Convulsions occurring due to meningitis, cerebral malaria or inflamed tonsils are not included. Febrile convulsions affect children aged between 2 and 4 years. Children with a positive family history of the condition are at an increased risk of the disorder.

Febrile convulsions should be treated actively as 40% of individuals who suffer from epilepsy have ever suffered from the condition in childhood. If untreated, febrile convulsions could lead to severe brain damage, subsequent learning disability, and or will require support from society for their survival.

- Teach first aid to prevent febrile convulsions in every child who has had at least one episode of febrile convulsions. First aid consists of tepid sponging the child in the face and the back of the head, combined with the use of paracetamol to control fever.
- The mother of any child with history of febrile convulsions should always be on the lookout to detect febrile illness.
- Ensure that a child suffers from febrile convulsions but not meningitis.
- Any child who has had at least one febrile convulsion before should be put on prophylactic phenobarbitone therapy.
- If prophylaxis is not indicated, the child should always be put on phenobarbitone during and for two weeks after an episode of febrile illness.

Note that Phenobarbitone may cause restlessness, over activity and other behaviour problems in children and the elderly, particularly those with brain damage. If this occurs, an alternative to Phenobarbitone such as Carbamazepine should be used. Where Carbamazepine is available, it should be used in place of Phenobarbitone in the dose of 50-100 mg at bedtime.

21
Morbid Jealousy

EMILIO OVUGA

Introduction

The term jealousy appeared as a disease entity in the medical literature in 1910 when it was introduced by Jasper. Thereafter the term acquired other names including amorous paranoia, morbid jealousy, pathologic jealousy and delusions of marital infidelity. The term delusion refers to the absolute conviction by an individual in an idea that is not true, and other member of the person's social group do not attest to it; a delusion is not alterable by reasonable arguments.

Normal jealousy

Jealousy as a normal human experience refers to the grief and pain experienced at the thought of losing a loved object to another person, such as a lover, a favored position among others in the community, or even a simple article such as a toy. The experience results from loss of self-esteem arising from the expected loss of the loved object, and is associated with feelings of enmity against the successful rival and self-criticism for one's loss.

Pathological jealousy

As an abnormal experience, jealousy is characterised by the abnormal belief that one's sexual partner is unfaithful and engages in secret sexual relationships with another person. The phenomenon may be associated with intense searching by the complainant for evidence; repeated interrogations and accusations; and violent quarrels to force a confession. Physical injuries may result and death may occur. Short of this the accused may lead a very miserable life in the face of the repeated violent accusations and the accompanying injuries. This form of abnormal jealousy affects more males than females but this difference may be culturally determined given that females are expected to be passive participants in sexual matters and relationships.

A second form of the disorder, reported usually by the husbands of sick wives, is characterised by excessive indulgence in sex by the affected woman. The basis of this problem is the belief by the sick woman that the husband has secret love affairs with other women, many of who may happen to be her own relatives and friends or the relatives of the husband. In order to keep the man satisfied and away from the alleged lovers of the husband, the woman begins to engage in excessive sexual relations with her husband. Unfortunately the more compliant the man is, the stronger the conviction of the woman and hence, the more she involves the husband in sexual activities. This problem may leave the man physically exhausted, psychologically miserable yet unable to defend himself against the wife's accusations. Interestingly such husbands are usually very humble, caring, and very supportive and it is probably these characteristics, which lead to the feelings of jealousy experienced by their wives.

Abnormal jealousy usually affects men aged over forty years, and it is most commonly caused by excessive use of alcohol, which interferes with sexual performance; the man typically blames the wife for his repeated failures that might have resulted in the loss of sexual drive in the wife, prompting the development of the delusion. Other causes include brain diseases such as resulting from blood vessel disease associated with normal ageing. The affected person usually has features of suspiciousness in their basic personality. On the other hand women who are affected by the problem usually suffer from conditions such as schizophrenia or manic depressive illness, which is characterised by episodes of elated mood, excitement, and unusual feelings of well-being, alternating with episodes of extreme sadness, misery, feeling of dejection and a desperate state of hopelessness.

Caution

It is important to note that morbid jealousy always assumes the guise of normal complaints between spouses in their marriage, and it becomes difficult to draw the line between what can be regarded as normal rather than pathological and requiring professional help. The difference here is qualitative as well as quantitative in nature. Qualitatively the abnormal complaints of infidelity are intense and many lead to coercive behaviour, which is often violent behind the closed curtains of marital affairs; there is usually no doubt in the mind of the complainant that he/she might be wrong; he or she is absolutely right about the unfaithfulness of the spouse! Quantitatively morbid jealousy leads to numerous interventions by family, elders and religious leaders within our cultural system to no avail; no amount of persuasion helps as the individual is absolutely right about the conduct of the spouse.

When excessive, complaints of marital infidelity leveled by any person against their spouse should be taken seriously, and professional advice sought to prevent misery in the home.

Management

The management of pathological jealousy usually begins late when the suspected victim has usually suffered severe emotional exhaustion and sometimes physical injury. Currently affected persons might come to the mental health professional through friends as a last resort, and a few might come through the courts as a result of assault on the suspected unfaithful spouse. In the end the affected spouse might also meet criteria to access professional care as much as the complainant. In the case of the victim, the problem might be post-traumatic stress disorder, and in the case of the complainant, assessment might lead to the underlying diagnosis.

- Care options following comprehensive history, physical examination, mental status assessment and biomedical investigations will include:
- Medication for the diagnosed underlying mental disorder
- Supportive psychotherapy
- Involvement of the social network as indicated

Prognosis may be guarded depending on the underlying factor. On the average complainants tend to adjust to, and live with their beliefs without taking steps against their spouses.

22
Personality Disorders

EMILIO OVUGA

Introduction

Personality disorders are a group of persistent stable and more or less permanent behavioural patterns of responding to a wide range of personal and social situations. They represent significant departures from the way the average person in a given culture perceives, thinks, feels and relates to other people in their community (WHO 1992). Personality disorders begin in childhood or early adolescence, continue into adulthood and usually persist throughout life and leads to distress and impairment (APA 1992) even though this may not appear obvious to people in the individual's social environment. Personality disorders are recognised as such if they are not due to another psychiatric disorder or the effect of alcohol dependence or abuse of other addictive substance. Remember though that personality disorder may be an additional diagnosis under Axis II in the multi-axial system of diagnosis. Thus the diagnosis of personality disorder may be made if its onset predates the onset of psychiatric disorder.

Personality disorders are clinically significant for practical reasons. They represent persistent expressions of an individual's inner world and experience, his or her characteristic lifestyle and mode of relating to people and the self under different situations. These behavioural patterns make it possible for predictions to be made about the likely type of response an affected person might make, or what type of mental health problem the person might develop given the experience of a stressful life event. This group of illnesses makes it harder for affected individuals to adapt to a variety of personal, social and environmental situations that require flexibility for harmonious relationships.

The Diagnostic and Statistical Manual of Mental Disorders of the American Psychological Association (APA 1992) lists over 10 different personality disorder types. Other personality types which were first described as such now appear as disorders under specific clinical disorder categories. Personality disorders do not exist within clear-cut boundaries and one individual may exhibit features of two or more types. In many situations individuals with personality disorder may not be recognised as such if they function normally within the expectations of their community. The exact prevalence of personality disorders is not known in Uganda as no population surveys have been conducted for this purpose. However, clinical experience suggests that 6% of patients with mental health problems receiving psychiatric care have one or other form of personality disorder. The proportion of personality disorders in prison populations is expected to be higher, and might be in the region of 10%. Personality disorder is a social and cultural construct, and the relative frequency of different types is determined by the culture in which one resides. Under normal clinical circumstances individuals with personality disorder rarely get to see the mental health care provider. For these reasons only four personality types will be described in this book. The four personality disorder types have been chosen because of their relative importance in shaping the behaviour of most cultures; they seem to be common to all cultures.

Paranoid Personality Disorder

The essential feature is a persistent and recurrent, often baseless, pattern of distrust and suspicion towards others. Individuals with this type of personality disorder strongly believe that they are the object of well planned harm, malice, plot, and exploitation. The individuals concerned interpret every statement, action or sign in the behaviour of other people as confirmation of their beliefs or their doubts of loyalty. Persons with this type of personality disorder persistently bear grudges against other people and are unforgiving of insults, failures, slights or mishaps. The commonest victims of paranoid personality are spouses, close friends or acquaintances, neighbors, workmates and business colleagues. If no evidence exists to justify their beliefs people with this disorder will craftily manipulate their social environment into carrying out the actions they want to see, and then use this as evidence of their beliefs. Individuals with paranoid personality disorder are always quick to react, accuse or seek redress, and they will more often than not overburden the criminal or civil justice system because of their unending complaints. In clinical practice paranoid personality commonly leads to the development of paranoid disorders such as paranoid schizophrenia, morbid jealousy, and paranoid psychosis secondary physical illness. In politics this type of personality disorder may breed tyranny and dictatorship.

Antisocial Personality Disorder

The essential feature of this disorder is the persistent violation of the rights of others and society. The disorder begins in early childhood or adolescence. Individuals with this type of personality disorder are deceitful and skillful at the manipulation of others in their social milieu. Persons with anti-social personality disorder appear not to conform to social norms with respect to lawful behaviour, repeatedly carry out actions that lead to their repeated arrest by the police or would be grounds for their appearance before their local council courts. People with anti-social personality are impulsive and do not plan, exhibit irritable aggression and fight often, are careless and do not care about their own safety or the safety of others, irresponsible and cannot retain jobs for any reasonable length of time or keep appointments, and lack ability to show remorse for any wrongs they may have caused. Instead, people with this type of personality will blame the rest of society for causing them troubles. Young people who will develop anti-social personality disorder in the future can be recognised using the following symptoms.

- Disciplinary problems both at home and school.
- Early use of alcohol and drugs of abuse
- Early involvement in indiscrete sexual behaviour
- Frequent fights with other children and peers
- Persistent lying, deceit
- Persistent theft
- Running away from home or other authority figures

Schizoid Personality Disorder

The essential feature of schizoid personality disorder is a persistent pattern of lack of interest in being part of their social groups, family or community. Individuals with this type of personality appear too interested in spending their time alone and are often described as "loners". They choose solitary life and do not appear to derive pleasure in the things that interest others in their social milieu. They do not appear to appreciate praises or criticisms and often exhibit emotional coldness, detachment or flat affective response. Schizoid personality disorder predisposes to the development of schizophrenia.

Histrionic Personality Disorder

The central feature of this type of personality disorder is excessive emotional reactivity and attention-seeking behaviour in a variety of social contexts. Individuals with this type of personality disorder often skillfully become the center of attraction in any group. Persons with histrionic personality are dramatic in their relationships with other people. They will often go out of their way to please others in the hope that they will receive a reward. If this fails their reaction can be embarrassingly disappointing to others, an effect that the individuals were up against. Histrionic personality disorder may predispose to depressive disorder or adjustment disorder with depressed mood. It is prevalent among members of the performing arts and politicians.

Narcissistic Personality Disorder

The main feature of this type of personality disorder is a persistent pattern of grandiosity, inflated self-image, a demanding need for admiration by others, and excessive pre-occupation with personal importance in the lives of others. The individual with this type of personality disorder will publicly proclaim that there is no other who parallels his or her in qualities, skills, and abilities and harshly devalues the contributions of others in public or communal life. People with narcissistic personality disorder believe that they are superior, special or unique and expect others to recognise them for their special contributions to their community and will repeatedly remind their audience with lengthy and tiring detail of their personal achievements in order to win and or sustain their admiration and loyalty. They are often deceitfully charming, kind, friendly, and polite when everything goes as they expect; they will often fish for praise and admiration. Persons with narcissistic personality are usually pre-occupied with wealth and property and hold an insatiable desire to own business and beat others in material possessions. However, when things do not go well for them and their sense of entitlement is not satisfied or snubbed, they become unreasonably puzzled and or furious. People with narcissistic personality disorder are particularly skillful in their use of other people to achieve their goals and will use all strategies including kidnapping, torture, murder and extortion if they have political or other means of power.

23
Problems in Sexual Function

Emilio Ovuga

Introduction

Sexual dysfunction is a disturbance in sexual desire and or the psychological and physical responses that constitute sexual functioning. There are several disorders of sexual function. However, the number of people who suffer from sexual dysfunction is not known due to lack of research data. Issues of sexual nature are regarded as personal and private in African culture, and this further accounts for the lack of information on how common the problem is. For practical purposes it may be said that the disorder is common, though it is rarely recognised and treated. Disorders of sexual function cause serious emotional distress, sometimes severe enough to lead to suicide or attempted suicide, strained marital relations or outright marital break-up. In this chapter the more common types of sexual disorder relevant to the cultures in Uganda are briefly described with an outline of management suggestions.

Causes of sexual dysfunction

Sexual dysfunction may be due to:

a) Physical disorders, e.g.
   - Hypertension
   - Diabetes mellitus
   - During the recovery phase of any acute physical illness
   - Poor functioning of the gonads, especially the testes in males

b) Alcohol abuse, medication, e.g. sedatives, anti-hypertensive medication

c) Mental disorder, most commonly depression, anxiety disorder

d) Strained marital relationships

e) Fear of infection, pregnancy, or physical injury during sexual intercourse

f) Inferiority feelings, fear of failure, fear of rejection

g) Strict discipline and religious upbringing

h) Rape and defilement

Types of sexual dysfunction

a) Lack of sexual desire is characterised by recurrent or persistent absence of or low levels of desire, interest or appetite for activity

b) Active avoidance of sexual contact is characterised by persistent or recurrent avoidance of any genital contact with sexual partner

c) Male erectile dysfunction is characterised by persistent or recurrent inability by a male to attain or sustain an erection long enough to complete sexual activity to the full satisfaction of both sexual partners

d) Inhibited female orgasm is characterised by recurrent or persistent inability of a female to reach the climax of sexual activity due to delays or absence of the climax

e) Inhibited male orgasm is recurrent or persistent delay in or absence of the male to reach sexual climax

f) Premature ejaculation is persistent or recurrent seminal emission with minimal sexual stimulation, or shortly after vaginal penetration and before the male wishes the occurrence of the emission

g) Dyspareunia is painful sexual intercourse in either a male or female

h) Vaginismus is persistent or recurrent spasms of the vaginal muscles that prevents vaginal penetration or free intercourse

Clinical presentation

Due to the problems stemming from cultural attitudes beliefs and practices problems in sexual life do not present as openly as they should, and indirect forms of communication may be used.

a) Reports of masturbation by a young male may indicate sexual dysfunction due to fear, shame, guilt or other negative beliefs about sexual activity; such a man will exhibit timid shy behaviour in the presence of females

b) Reports of fear by a young woman of culturally appropriate advances made by any young man towards her

c) Vague and chronic headache, which may be associated with cramps in the muscles and with or without fever throughout the day

d) Chronic pelvic pain, low back ache in a woman

e) Chronic genital discharge in a woman

f) Reports to elders in the family by a married woman over the sexual conduct of the husband

g) Complaints of infertility

h) Direct complaints of lack of desire for sex, of impotence, and of inability to ejaculate or to reach orgasm

i) Disagreements, arguments or quarrels over very minor issues in the home

j) Alcohol abuse. Note that the role of alcohol abuse in sexual life may be both ways; it may cause the disorder but it may also result from the disorder as a management method.

Investigations

The aims of investigations are to identify any physical causes to the sexual dysfunction, determine if psychological factors, whether personal or marital may be responsible, and to determine social factors that may be responsible. Investigations that may be conducted include the following:

- 24-hour-urine analysis for male and female hormones
- Any laboratory tests suggested by results of clinical interview and physical examination
- Routine laboratory tests including full haemogram, urinalysis and liver function tests.

Management approaches

Since the causes of sexual dysfunction are many and varied, it may not be easy to provide appropriate care without first understanding the factors responsible for the dysfunction. In general the appropriate methods of care in primary care fall under four categories.

- **Talk therapy** to address identified psychological personal issues that interfere with normal sex life; it may be better to involve both partners at this stage if the factors in the dysfunction are thought to be marital in nature.
- **Behavioural therapy** that was developed by Masters and Johnson in the United States of America teaches practical steps to sexual behaviour; the technique has proved effective in the Ugandan context.
- **Medication** to treat any physical condition thought to be responsible for sexual dysfunction. If the main reason for the dysfunction is failure of the testes hormone therapy may be indicated. Most commonly a drug may be used to improve blood circulation in the penis to improve the quality of sexual activity by the middle-aged or elderly man.
- **Surgical intervention** using appropriate appliances may be used to sustain erection if no psychological or medical condition is found.

Managing sexual dysfunction is complex and is governed not only by cultural and social factors but also ethical issues. When in doubt refer to a senior colleague.

24
Forensic Psychiatry

EMILIO OVUGA

Introduction

Forensic psychiatry is a branch of psychiatry that is concerned with the assessment, investigations, diagnosis and treatment of mental disorders among three broad categories of individuals:

- Individuals who are alleged to have committed an offence and face prosecution
- Convicted prisoners who develop mental illness in the course of serving their sentence
- Individuals who have not committed any offence but whose mental capacity is in question.

Under existing mental health legislation in Uganda it is not expected that the primary health care provider will provide this service. It is however advisable that the primary health care provider knows something about prisoners' mental health needs for the purpose of early and appropriate referrals to centers where a psychiatrist or other mental health professional is available. This chapter describes the types of services offered in forensic psychiatry.

Individual facing prosecution

The individual who faces prosecution may come to the attention of the psychiatrist on the following grounds:

a) The Police might notice signs of mental disorder in the individual in their custody

b) The Presiding Magistrate or Judge may observe signs of mental disorder

c) Relatives might have raised the issue of mental disorder

d) The prisoner might personally report history of treatment for psychiatric disorder.

e) The suspect might plead insane during court proceedings

Under any of the above grounds the Magistrate may order an assessment and or observation of the individual to ascertain:

Whether the individual is mentally disordered

a) The ability of the individual to stand trial if he/she is mentally disordered

b) Whether the accused is criminally responsible for the offence he/she is charged with

To answer each of the three questions above the psychiatrist with his/her team will usually:

- Hospitalise the person concerned for the purpose of observations and possible treatment or attend to the matter on an out-patient basis
- Take a "full psychiatric history" including the history of previous episodes of illness and treatment
- Order an observation of the person by nursing staff and other health care providers on daily basis
- Conduct laboratory, psychological and social investigations
- Make a report to the Magistrate who will then decide on the best course of action on the basis of the psychiatric report

Criminal responsibility

Criminal responsibility is a legal concept, which refers to the extent to which an individual can be held liable for his/her offence. A clinical test of responsibility (Criteria for criminal responsibility) (Ovuga, 1991) may be used to determine whether an individual is responsible for an offence or not. See the criteria in table 1.

Table 24.1: Criteria for criminal responsibility

Criteria for Criminal Responsibility (CCR)	Score
1. Offence required careful ***planning***	
2. Offence was unrelated to ***symptoms*** of mental disorder	
3. Identifiable ***motive*** for the crime was not the product of mental disorder	
4. Mental ***capacity*** at the time of the crime was unimpaired or did not impair rational judgment	
5. ***Amnesia*** if present is incongruent with relevant key features of the crime and mental state	

Score each item 1 for a "Yes" response and 0 for a "No" response. The maximum possible score is 5. A score of 3 or more indicates that the individual is probably responsible for an alleged crime. Note that amnesia indicates an organic mental disorder. However, it is possible for certain forms of partial seizure to occur in the absence of amnesia. Other forms of mental disorder, e.g. major depression and paranoid disorder may lead to the execution of well planned crimes. An act becomes a crime if it can be proved that the individual formed intent to execute the act. Intent in this sense is closely related to the question of motive, which is one of the criteria to determine criminal responsibility (See table 1 above). A score less than 3 on the CCR (individual is not responsible) is well likely to be associated with poor mental capacity to form intent. Table 24.2 below lists the elements of mental capacity to form intent. It may be advisable to use tables 24.1 and 24.2 together deciding on the issue of criminal responsibility.

Table 24.2: Elements of capacity to form intent

Elements of mental capacity to form intent in commission of an offence
Appreciate the nature and quality of one's behaviour
Appreciate the wrongfulness of one's behaviour
Appreciate the likely consequences of one's behaviour on other people
Refrain from engaging in any wrongful act
Act in conformity with established societal code of conduct

Ability to stand trial

An individual will not be expected to have an ability to stand trial if the following observations apply to him/her.

- Mentally ill with active signs of mental disorder
- Lacks ability to understand court proceedings

When an accused person is found unable to stand trial on grounds of active mental illness, the psychiatrist may recommend that the individual receives the relevant treatment for the mental disorder. After full recovery the individual may then be able to stand trial. However, individuals who suffer from severe psychotic illness, such as schizophrenia sometimes relapse into active illness if their case is not disposed off soon after a recommendation is made. In these circumstances it would be prudent to make a recommendation that will help the trial court to use its discretion to dispose of the case early.

Convicted prisoner

When a prisoner who is serving a sentence falls ill he/she may be referred to a mental hospital under the Magistrates Court Act for assessment, observation and treatment. Unfortunately, under existing laws such an individual will not be excused from serving his/her prison sentence on ground of mental illness and he/she will be released at the end of the prison sentence.

Aims of management in forensic work

Forensic work aims to achieve the following objectives:

- Diagnose to form the basis for treatment and or recommendation to court
- Make a report and submit it to court
- Rehabilitate as part of management
- Promote acceptance of the individual in his/her community
- Resettle the individual back in his/her community
- Promote after care following discharge from the courts and hospital

A non-prisoner whose mental capacity is queried

Various reasons lead to request the mental health professional to assess and report on the mental capacity of individuals. The most common source of requests is from family members and other relatives. The person in question is likely to be elderly and his/her estate may be at the center of the request, a spouse caught up in a legal battle with the partner, an employee who is facing dismissal or retirement from his/her post on medical grounds. See chapter on report writing.

Providing mental health services to prisoners

Although it is possible to provide services to prisoners there is no system that supports the service. The Penal Code Act presumes that an accused person is sane until proved otherwise. To prove an accused person insane requires that the issue of insanity be raised by someone in the first place. As such the majority of prisoners in Uganda have no access to mental health services at all till it is too late. Research among remand prisoners (Adaku, 2005) indicated that one in every two remand prisoners had some form of mental illness though none of these had received any form of health assessment. Moreover many of these individuals had been mentally ill before and some had received treatment for their mental disorder previously. It is therefore possible that convicted prisoners who develop mental illness while in prison might receive medical care before their trial begins if this service were available.

The provision of mental health services in prison requires education of the police, prison authorities and the judiciary to raise their awareness to this potential need. When the need is established, assessment and medication might be provided to those in need, most probably within the prison environment. This will then require the development of a drug administration, monitoring and evaluation system to ensure that required drugs are utilized appropriately within the policy framework for the provision of health care to prisoners. Assessment for the purpose of determining criminal responsibility or for the issuance of reports should be left to the psychiatrist and any such requests should be referred accordingly.

Table 24.3: Annex

Format for Forensic Psychiatric Report	
Identification • Name, qualifications, position held, place of work **Background to report** • Basis for the report • About who? • At whose request? • Purpose of report **Personal identification of the person concerned** • Name, sex, age, marital status, residence, occupation, religion	**Introduction** • Legal status or otherwise of the person concerned • Circumstances of subject matter, i.e. what occasioned the request for a report? • Sources of data/information • How were data/information gathered? E.g. interviews, observations, laboratory tests, psychological investigations, social investigations, special investigations etc.
Circumstances of the crime or nature of other basis for requesting for a report Full description of any mental disorder • Current illness • Features of illness at the time of crime or relevant to basis of request for report • Description of all previous episodes of mental disorder if any **Personal development history** • Pre-natal, natal, post-natal history • Early childhood history: o First month of life o First year of life o Years 1-5 o Mid-childhood o Adolescence	**Personal development** • Reaction to birth of siblings • Reaction to visitors, strangers • Reaction to sickness at home • Reaction to quarrels at home • Reaction to first date, first day out of home, first day at school, first day of menarche or puberty, first day visiting other relatives, etc • Rape, violence, bullying, child abuse, war **Social history** • Ability to make friends; who initiates? • Education • Employment • Marital status • Birth of first child and subsequent offspring

• E.g. Important events that an be recalled • Neurotic behaviors e.g. temper tantrums, sleep disorders, enuresis, problems with eating, avoidance behavior, childhood speech problems, special fears, alcohol/ illicit drug use • Disciplinary problems • Anxiety disorders • Childhood mood disorders • Other mental disorder • Febrile convulsions; other neurologic problems in childhood	**Family history** • Mental illness, suicide behavior, alcohol/drug abuse, epilepsy, crime • Family discord, separation, bereavement **Premorbid personality** • Antisocial, conduct disorder, paranoid, borderline personality disorders **Physical assessment, laboratory and special investigations** Results of these relevant to the required report, especially opinion, and recommendations

Opinion

- Intent
- Capacity
- Will
- Motive
- Sum these up in relation to crime vis-a-vis mental disorder
- Prognosis
- Response to treatment so far Recommendations
- Future care needs
- Social support
- Risk assessment for crime/violence, etc
- Disposal: quote relevant sections of Acts

25
Somatoform Disorders (Psychosomatic Disorders)

EMILIO OVUGA

Introduction

Somatoform disorders were previously known as psychosomatic disorders. These are physical complaints arising from mental stress. Although the person has physical complaints, it is hard or impossible to detect a physical cause. They may have many symptoms or vague symptoms e.g. pains and aches all over the body. They may have a minor disease but this does not account for the numerous or vague physical complaints.

The mechanism through which psychological response to stressful life events manifest in physical symptoms is not clearly understood. It has been postulated that different individuals have different susceptibilities to respond to the challenges of daily living through the automatic activation of neurological, endocrine, biochemical and or metabolic systems in the body to mobilise sufficient resources to cope with personal life events.

Conditions, which commonly present as psychosomatic disorders are:

- Asthma
- Peptic ulcers
- Essential Hypertension
- Arthritis
- Ulcerative Colitis
- Eczema
- Migraine

Potential symptom patterns

Symptoms of somatoform disorder may be related to the physiological functioning of specific organ systems, and may be influenced by the patient's level of understanding of the functions of different parts of the body. In this way somatoform disorders can be grouped according to symptoms related to abnormal functioning of specific systems of the stressed body.

Individuals who tend to respond to stressors in their lives with the activation of the respiratory system will exhibit hyperventilation and or difficulty in breathing. Those who respond with Generalised activation of the loco motor system might complain of Generalised aches and muscle pains including headache.

Other individuals might present with palpitations, and or changes in heartbeat including sensation of missed heartbeat. Persons who suffer from somatoform disorder seem to be easily suggestible to specific symptom patterns that resemble the symptoms of illness in a relative or family member who might have suffered from or died with. Somatoform disorders may mask depression or anxiety disorder.

It has been suggested that the symptoms of somatoform disorder represent a method of communicating psychological distress, a method of communication that is culturally and socially acceptable, and which enhances access to health care and fits in the medical model of health care. Specific examples of common medical symptoms that might fall under this category are asthma, eczema, arthritis, hypertension, peptic ulcer and migraine headache.

Example 1

A 14-year-old schoolboy presented with episodes of vomiting, abdominal pain and general weakness, which led to repeated episodes of hospital consultation and days off from school. Associated loss of appetite led to weight loss and deterioration of general health. It was noted that the episodes of illness recurred within one to two days of the boy's return to school. It turned out the boy was worried that he might be ill with AIDS as suggested by a naughty school-mate because the 14-year-old boy looked too small and frail for his age. The parents of the boy lived apart and he was worried about this.

Example 2

One day a young woman in her twenties was brought to a rural clinic in southwestern Uganda. She had several complaints that included backache, pains in the chest and abdomen and aches in the muscles. The patient produced a polythene bag full of drugs that she had received from various clinics, but which she refused to take saying that she did not think she needed the drugs. Physical examination revealed nothing wrong and psychological oriented interview and assessment revealed that the woman's boy friend had died two years earlier. She believed that the boy friend died of AIDS and was therefore worried about the possibility of dying soon. Serological assessment for HIV showed that the girl was not infected, and this was all that she needed to regain her health and hopes in life. The woman is happily employed.

Example 3

A 34-year-old mother complained that she was no longer able to care for her baby and reported that her right arm was both weak and heavy. She complained that she could not sleep well, had no appetite and felt tired most of the time. She constantly thought about dying and wished that God would make her die in her sleep. The woman reported that her problems were due to her husband who had made life difficult for her. Physical examination of the arm showed no abnormality even though the woman did exhibit obvious effort in trying to use it.

Management

Treatment of somatoform disorder produces variable results. Therapeutic approaches that have been reported to yield good results are antidepressant therapy with tricyclic antidepressants, and supportive psychotherapy. In primary health care psychiatry, the establishment of a trusting relationship with the patient to foster an understanding of the patient's life situation and experiences is likely to enhance good clinical outcomes in the medical management of somatoform disorders.

26
Psychiatric Emergencies

Emilio Ovuga

A psychiatric emergency is a situation in mental health requiring immediate attention to avoid possible death, self-harm or harm to other people. Psychiatric emergencies require immediate attention as they pause a danger to the person, community and or property. It is therefore imperative that Health workers remain alert all the time to be able to protect the patient, communities and property from harm or destruction.

Disorders and situations causing psychiatric emergencies

Psychiatric emergencies usually occur in the context of mental disorders, which can be recognised whether at home or in hospital. The clinical condition of the patient is a key determinant as to whether a condition is an emergency or not. The following are mental disorders that may be associated with psychiatric emergency.

- Major depressive disorder
- Acute organic psychosis (delirium and delirium tremens may cause exhaustion, dehydration, harm)
- Postpartum psychosis (may lead to infanticide)
- Schizophrenia (paranoid schizophrenia; schizophrenic excitement)
- Manic excitement (exhaustion, dehydration)
- Personality disorder, e.g. anti-social personality disorder, paranoid personality disorder may lead to harm to others
- Drug intoxication may lead to harm
- Delinquency
- Post-ictal confusion in epilepsy
- Chronic organic brain syndrome
- Aggressive psychopaths
- Situational; psychiatric emergencies may be triggered by specific situations that may or may not be related to a person's mental disorder.

General Principles of Management of Psychiatric Emergencies

1. The patient should be attended to as soon as possible and relatives should be reassured.
2. Panic on the part of the staff worries the relatives more and may worsen the patients' symptoms, thus the need to be calm.
3. Initial treatment should focus on providing relief of acute and distressing symptoms. Treatment of the cause of the emergency can wait till later.
4. Some conditions have similar symptoms. It is important to differentiate between these conditions so that correct treatment may be given for the appropriate disorder.
5. Note that the psychiatric emergencies can reoccur, therefore, it is important that health education talks be given to the patient, relative, workmates/classmates and where possible follow-up for prevention of such recurrences.

A health worker should look out for the following conditions:-

- Attempted suicide
- Aggressive and violent behaviour (Acute psychotic states)
- Status epilepticus (this is not a mental disorder but a neurological condition, which is best managed by a physician)
- Rape and defilement
- Child disappearing from home

Suicide behaviour

Suicide behaviour is a spectrum of human behaviour that may lead to a person killing him or herself, and comprises of the following elements

- Wish to die
- Wish to commit suicide
- Communication of the intention to commit suicide
- Making suicide plan
- Execution of suicide plan
- Suicide attempt
- Completed suicide

Prevalence

80 people commit suicide every hour worldwide. Up to 40% of the general population experience the wish to die at least once in their lifetime. The World Health Organisation estimates that by the year 2020, there will be one suicide every 20 seconds and one suicide attempt every 1-2 seconds (Bertolote, 2001).

Suicide is common in Uganda though the rate may vary from region to region, and from sub-county to sub-county. In one sub-county in Adjumani district the rate of suicide has been estimated at 99 per 100,000 inhabitants in 2003, and the rate of suicide attempt was estimated to be 518 per 100,000 inhabitants in 2002. In 2004 the estimated rate for suicide in the whole district of Adjumani was 49.6 per 100,000 inhabitants and that of attempted suicide, 50.1 per 100,000 inhabitants. At least 15% of the population in Uganda have a previous history of suicide attempt (Ovuga, 2005) and 16% of the adult population report the experience of suicide behaviour in the past year (Kanarukara et al, 2004).

Aetiology

- 90% of suicides occur within the context of a mental disorder, particularly depression; suicide behaviour can occur in the context of any mental disorder.
- Difficulties in interpersonal relationships.
- Adverse socio-economic circumstances.
- Chronic physical illness, e.g. cancer, HIV/AIDS, congestive cardiac failure.

Attempted suicide

Suicide attempt may occur in the following conditions and situation:

1. Depressive illness
2. Schizophrenia
3. Panic (anxiety) disorder
4. Chronic organic brain syndrome

5. Under the influence of alcohol and/or drugs
6. Manic disorder
7. Post-traumatic stress disorder
8. Following rape/defilement

Common methods used for committing suicide

- Ingesting poison
- Jumping from a height, hanging and inhaling poisonous gases.
- Drowning
- Self starvation.

High risk Factors

- Negative ideas about life - hopelessness, lack of meaning in life
- Feeling of social rejection, abandonment, lack of social support system
- Presence of mental illness, particularly depression
- Presence of suicide behaviour
- Previous history of suicide attempt
- Family history of suicide attempt or completed suicide
- Presence of general medical illness

Other Risk Factors

- Sex - more males commit suicide than females
- Age - those aged more than 44 years tend to commit rather than attempt suicide.
- Alcohol - concomitant alcohol or other drug abuse raise the risk of suicide.
- Loss of rational thinking - the loss of rational thinking, as occurs in delirium, schizophrenia or manic excitement raises the risk of suicide.
- The presence of interpersonal difficulties including marital difficulties in Uganda is associated with high risk of successful suicide.
- Evidence of organised plan is associated with high risk of successful suicide.

- Recent loss of status, role, and esteem in social relationships predisposes to successful suicide.

  Poverty and unemployment - suicide is a disease of poverty.
- Circumstances of a previous or planned suicide bid - if the individual attempted, or plans to carry out a suicide act when rescue was/is unlikely, then the risk of successful suicide is very high.
- Timing - most successful suicides occur after midnight or mid-morning when rescue from a suicide bid is unlikely.
- Method - the choice of a hard method such as hanging points to a high risk of successful suicide.
- Communication of suicide wish or suicide intent is one of the most powerful predictors of successful suicide. Remember, though, that communication of suicide intent may be intended to elicit last minute help from close social contacts; the motive of communication should therefore be evaluated adequately. The communication of suicide intent may be direct or subtle.
  - Direct communication: "If you think that I am not the head of this home, I will leave this world for you."
  - Indirect communication: "I am fed up with life. I wish I were not born."
- Suicide note - the presence of a suicide note for a previous attempt, or plan to leave a suicide note before executing a planned suicide act is associated with a high suicide risk.
- The absence of dependents or lack of specific responsibility for the welfare of other family members carries a high risk of suicide.
- Evaluation of failed suicide act - an individual who is disappointed with the failure of a suicide bid may attempt suicide again.

Assessing suicide risk

A highly suicidal patient:

- Is severely depressed or has overt signs of florid psychosis.
- Has attempted or tried to attempt suicide before coming to you.
- Has an urgent wish to die, possibly within a week or so; natural death is too far.

- Has an active plan for implementing suicide plan.
- Will feel disappointed if suicide bid fails.
- May have communicated the suicide intention to some one else.

Remember that suicide risk remains substantial up to three months after apparent clinical recovery. Suicide prevention measures should therefore remain in force and the patient should be monitored regularly for suicide potential. The best precaution to take in suicide prevention and suicide risk assessment is to detect suicide potential proactively in every high risk patient.

Management of suicide behaviour

- Detect suicide behaviour in every patient with clinical interview. Up to 46% of the general population have suicide ideation (Ovuga et al, 2005).
- Determine the risk of suicide occurring.
- Detect the presence of a psychiatric disorder, particularly depression, or chronic general medical illness or psycho-social stressors.
- Develop treatment and suicide prevention plan with patient and carer.
- Educate the patient and carer about suicide behaviour.
- Suicide behaviour is a normal human experience.
- Suicide behaviour can be treated.
- Talking about death, dying and suicide helps people to drop the suicide idea.
- Start medication for appropriate psychiatric disorder.
- Discuss the prevention of suicide behaviour with colleague in-charge of general medical care (as appropriate).
- Enter into a contract with the patient so that he/she can contact carer, friend, or yourself in case he/she experiences the suicide urge.
- Start cognitive therapy aimed at reducing the patient's irrational and negative ideas, beliefs, and attitudes and, at teaching the patient effective problem-solving skills as described in item 10 below.
- Help the patient solve or cope with interpersonal problems or current and ongoing psychosocial stressor. Gently guide the patient to :

- Narrate the nature of his/her current and ongoing life difficulties.
- Describe his/her previous, current and ongoing psycho-social stressors.
- Evaluate the meaning and significance of his/her difficulties and psychosocial stressors In relation to his/her aspirations, plans and hopes in life.
- Develop a hierarchy of his/her usual responses to life stressors.
- Evaluate the effectiveness of each of these responses.

  Develop alternative responses and strategies to solve his/her difficulties.
- Develop homework for the patient to carry out.
- Evaluate the outcome of the implementation of home work assignments and identify problems and obstacles the patient encountered; discuss how the patient could get round the identified problems, etc.
- Dispense drugs on weekly basis only till the risk of suicide has substantially been removed.
- If in doubt refer to the psychiatrist, psychologist or professional counsellor early.

Prevention of suicide behaviour

The prevention of suicide should be the task of every health worker. The prevalence of suicide behaviour can be reduced through:

- Early detection of suicide ideas among patients.
- Early detection of depression.
- Effective treatment of disorders associated with suicide.
- Improve prescription habits that promote safety in psychotropic drug use.
- Improving general socio-economic situation of communities.

Caution in case of suicide behaviour

- Every suicide attempt should be taken seriously as a successful attempt may follow thereafter.
- The patient is often unmanageable in an out-patient setting, therefore, requires hospitalisation.

- The patient should be under close observation; potentially harmful materials such as drugs, sharp objects should be removed.
- If suspected to have taken poison, close observation and antidote for poison should be given.
- When the patients life is no longer in immediate danger from suicide, a health worker should talk to the patient to understand the reasons why the patient was attempting suicide.
- A health worker should adopt an understanding rather than a punitive or judgmental working attitude.
- The underlying psychotic disorders e.g. depression or schizophrenia should be managed appropriately.

Aggressive and violent behaviour

Psychiatric emergency may take the form of aggressive behaviour, which may be unprovoked and is usually directed at family members. In this case the aggression may be in response to delusions that the victim is behind the sick person's continued illness or in protest against being taken to traditional healers or being locked up in a room alone. Frequently aggression may be provoked by members of the general public through insults directed at the mentally ill who may be passing by.

- Schizophrenia
- Acute organic syndrome especially alcohol intoxication, drug intoxication and delirium.

Management of aggressive behaviour

- In the case of the hospitalised patient do not take him/her by surprise, explain all the procedures you are going to do; assure the individual of his/her security
- It is important for a health worker not to become frightened or excited as this may reduce the effectiveness of any measures taken and interfere with finding a rational solution to a problem.
- There should be quick organised intervention to avoid injury to self and others, however, if you are alone seek help from others.

- A health worker should try to understand why a patient is aggressive before resorting to restraining methods.
- Enough human resources should be readily available.
- Be aware of the patient with aggression and show them that you are in control of the situation.
- In case of an armed patient, he should be disarmed without causing harm. During the process, do not all talk at once, let the person with the best relationship with the aggressive/violent individual do the talking in a calm and convincing manner.
- Never approach an aggressive mental patient alone.
- Use minimal restraint when necessary and discontinue when it is no longer necessary.
- Once the incident is over, follow up the patient to establish the possible cause of the behaviour.
- In case of organic brain syndrome, identify the physical cause and manage it accordingly. This type of patient requires extra care for which you should refer to (Unit 6.1 organic mental disorder) for detailed appropriate management.

Status Epilepticus

This a repeated attacks of generalised, tonic, clonic seizures without gaining consciousness in between. These may be caused by

- Sudden withdraw of anti epileptic drugs
- Infections
- Sudden stressful situations
- Starvation
- Excessive exhaustion
- Hormonal changes.

Management of status epilepticus

- Remove the patient from danger
- Loosen tight clothing
- Do not restrain the jerking

- Clear airway
- Do not give anything by mouth
- Place the patient in lateral position
- Refer to hospital for further management including investigations within 12 hours.

Caution in case of status epilepticus

Do not place anything between teeth during the attack, as this may injure the patients' gums.

Drugs in status epilepticus

- Diazepam 10 mg rectally (See details in the chapter on epilepsy)

Rape and defilement

Rape is defined as having sexual (carnal) knowledge of a woman without her consent. Defilement refers to having sexual relations with a female person under the age of 18 years. Though rape and defilement may also involve males and boys as victims of both adult women and men much of the attention remains focused on women and girls as victims of men; note also that adult women as perpetrators of the rape and defilement of women and girls has hardly been reported in the local press in Uganda. Apart from the physical injuries inflicted on the survivor, there are associated emotional and psychosocial effects of the trauma. However, whereas the physical injuries are given due attention the emotional and psychosocial sequelae are not taken care of though these often lead to short and long-term mental health effects on victims.

Physical effects of rape and defilement

- Injuries/bruises of the private and/other parts.
- Bleeding excessively.
- Infection, HIV/Syphilis/gonorrhea.
- Unwanted pregnancy.

Psychological effects of rape and defilement

- Fear and anxiety

- Depression
- Stigma
- Self guilt/blame
- Sleeplessness due to nightmares
- Re-experiencing the event rape
- Numbing of emotions
- Worthlessness, hopelessness and helplessness
- Feeling dirty
- May develop obsessive compulsive behaviour
- They may develop fear of the men in the case of women victims

Management of rape and defilement

It should be a comprehensive package, which involves:

- Counseling by experienced counsellor
- Respect for confidentiality
- Treating physical complications such as injuries and infections
- Follow up and home visiting
- In case of pregnancy refer to appropriate counsellor
- Ensure protection of the survivor from future abuse through life-skills training.

SECTION III

Child and Adolescent Mental Health

27
Mental Disorders in Children and Adolescents

GRACE NAKASI

Introduction

Half of the world's population is made up of children and adolescents. It is estimated that up to 20% of children and adolescents suffer from some form of mental disorder requiring treatment. A proportion of children with emotional problems will grow into adults carrying along with them any emotional problem that might not have been adequately managed. Promoting the mental health of children and adolescents is therefore equivalent to promoting the mental health of the world's entire population.

However the effective treatment and control of mental disorders in childhood and adolescence are hampered by attitudinal and conceptual problems. For example even though the need for psychiatric intervention might be obvious in the case of an individual child or adolescence, such intervention might not be provided in the often mistaken belief that the child or adolescent's symptoms are due to the normal process of growing up or normal response to social situation, that the emotional problem will naturally resolve, or the child or adolescent is simply being lazy, naughty or disobedient.

Psychiatric problems in childhood and adolescence may be symptoms of a dysfunctional social environment in which the child lives and the successful outcome of psychiatric intervention in the case of a given child or adolescent requires careful assessment of each clinical problem in which a child or adolescent is involved.

Untreated emotional or behavioural disorder may result in the poor development of the child or adolescent, inability to receive education, subsequent underachievement in life, poor future lifelong quality of life and dependency on other people for survival, crime, and drug abuse or dependence.

Common Childhood and Adolescent Emotional and Behavioural Disorders

Emotional and other psychiatric disorders commonly encountered in Uganda include the following:

- Depressive disorder
- Anxiety disorders
- Phobias
- Obsessive compulsive disorders
- Conversion disorders
- Conduct disorder
- Attention deficit and hyperactivity disorder
- Learning disability
- Adolescent substance abuse
- The emotional effects of HIV/AIDS
- Adolescent suicide

Common Causes of Emotional and Behaviour Disorders in Uganda

Several factors often operate leading to the onset of childhood and adolescent emotional and behavioural problems in Uganda and these include:

- General psychosocial stressors in the life of the child's family
- Family instability due to problems that affect the relationship of one parent to the other parent
- General socio-economic difficulties affecting the child or adolescent's family
- Poor neighbourhood with overcrowding, crime, delinquency and drug and substance abuse
- Parental or significant other care-giver loss due to separation or death
- The effects of social unrest, armed conflict and war
- Genetic predisposition – family history of mental disorder
- Brain injury during childbirth, head injury, or infection involving the brain
- Malnutrition and other nutritional disorders, e.g. childhood thyroid deficiency state
- Childhood HIV/AIDS

From childhood the common causes are:

1. Before birth
   - Syphilis
   - German measles
   - Injuries to mother
   - Attempted unsuccessful abortion
   - Poor feeding mother
   - Drug abuse of the mother e.g. alcohol
   - Hereditary.

2. During delivery
   - Prolonged labour
   - Complicated labour

3. Assisted delivery
   - Forceps
   - Vacuum extraction

4. After delivery
   - Repeated convulsions
   - Infectious diseases – tetanus, measles, meningitis, infections of the brain.

5. Environmental
   - Violence in the home
   - Frustrations
   - Family disintegration
   - Poor family relationships
   - Conflicts e.g. civil strife
   - Sexual, physical and emotional abuse
   - Loss of parents
   - Malnutrition (poor feeding)
   - Mental illness of parents or principal care taker.

Anxiety Disorder

An anxiety disorder is characterised by an unexplained fear that has persisted for at least three weeks. A child who suffers from an anxiety disorder may exhibit excessive fear of the dark, fear to sleep alone, fear to be left alone, may experience nightmares, or fear for personal safety or the safety of parent or other significant person in the family; the child may exhibit excessive dread for potential separation from parent or significant other care-taker. The child may be withdrawn, avoid situations that he or she fears, behave younger than his or her usual age, appear worried and lack concentration or interest in usual activity including academic work leading to poor performance at school. Health status may deteriorate, the child may lose weight and the need for health care may dramatically increase due to physical symptoms such as headache, dizziness, palpitations, tremors, sweating, central abdominal pain, nausea and vomiting.

Depressive disorder

Depressive disorder in childhood usually has the same general features as in adults, and it is characterised by depressed mood, social withdrawal, apathy, loss of interest in usual activities, irritability, loss of appetite, poor sleep, lack of energy, and overall poor health status. The child or adolescent may run away from home, become disobedient, live rough, perform poorly at school and or begin to use alcohol and drugs in the company of peers. Severe depression may, as in adults, be associated with ideas of hopelessness, pessimism, worthlessness, and suicidal thoughts.

Adolescent suicide

The phenomenon of adolescent suicide is similar to that in adults, and is characterised by the child or adolescent feeling that his or her situation is hopeless, the future is dark and empty, his or her life is worthless, and that his or her real hope lies in suicide. Suicidal adolescents or children are often regarded as being impulsive, exhibit a lot of aggression and lack confidence in those who may be trying to help them. The family background of suicidal children and adolescents may be characterised by social dysfunction, early separation from parent, alcohol abuse, child neglect, family history of mental illness, family history of suicide, and family history of criminal behaviour. The suicidal child or adolescent may threaten suicide before taking his or her life, though such prior warning is often ignored. Suicidal children or adolescents in Uganda often succeed though actual figures for successful suicide rate among them is not available. The single most significant warning sign of potential suicide in a child or adolescent is a warning of the event along with signs of

Phobia

A phobia is an anxiety disorder characterised by irrational fear of an object (e.g. insect, feather), or of a situation (e.g. fear of being left alone at home, fear of going out of home alone, fear of a crowd or fear of travelling by car or bus).

Obsessive compulsive disorder

An obsession is the experience of a senseless, repetitive, or unpleasant thought, imagination, wishes or fantasies that the child experiences against his or her wish and tries unsuccessfully to keep out of his or her mind. A compulsion is a repetitive action that the child might carry out against his or her wish, such as repetitively washing the hands, walking in and out the door repeatedly for a fixed number of times before finally going to school. A compulsion is usually linked to an obsession, which precedes it, thus the name obsessive compulsive disorder. For example on seeing the droppings of chicken a child felt that his mouth was contaminated with dirt. As a result the child constantly spat saliva endlessly in order to expel germs from his mouth.

Conversion disorder

A conversion disorder, previously known as hysteria, is an anxiety disorder in which the child presents with altered functioning of part of the body in response to an anxiety-arousing situation. Common forms of conversion disorder are sudden blindness, dumb-deafness, and paralysis of one limb or loss of sensory functioning over part of the body, the assumption of strange gait, or inability to swallow even liquids. The apparent loss of function of part of the adolescent or child's body has no valid disorder. Conversion disorder is common in girls' schools, and is often triggered among many by the onset of a physical symptom associated with an often trivial febrile illness affecting a girl of dominant character at school; the influence of ghosts may be blamed. On some occasions conversion symptoms in an adolescent girl may be accompanied by severe regression in behaviour to as young as the stage of suckling.

Attention Deficit and Hyperactivity Disorder

This is a disorder characterised by severe disruption of attention along with over activity. Attention deficit and hyperactivity disorder is thought to result from trivial brain damage that the child might have sustained during childbirth. The child with the disorder cannot sit still or remain at one place for any length of time, is always on the go and everywhere, and fears no dangers, climbing and playing dangerously with household objects. Due to the disruption of attention, the child cannot concentrate and has poor memory for most things that happen to him or her and may have severe learning difficulty. The affected child may engage in anti-social behaviour, exhibiting temper tantrums with aggressive behaviour including fighting other children over trivial matters. The child's behaviour naturally exhausts family members who spend considerable amount of their time protecting and guarding the child against accidental self-harm. The disorder is more common among boys than girls. It begins early in childhood and may continue into adulthood in one out of every three children affected. The outcome for this condition is crippling for those in whom it persists beyond puberty, implying lifelong dependence on others for personal livelihood and survival.

Conduct Disorder

Conduct disorder is characterised by a repeated pattern of behaviour, which is disapproved by society and includes stealing, running away from home or school, destruction of property, setting fire to property, sexually indiscrete behaviour including promiscuity, and use of alcohol and illicit drugs, disobedience and resistance to authority both at home and at school. Conduct disorder is caused by multiple interacting factors that include family disharmony and frequent family quarrels, the influence of bad peer groups, poor parent-child relationships, poor teacher-child relationships and poor and cruel disciplinary methods employed by parents or other authority figures. Other factors include low social class, large family with inadequate individual care from parents and the absence of a father figure. A child with conduct disorder is touchy, has temper tantrums, quarrels with other family members or other individuals.outside the family, argues with parents and blames other people for his or her hardships almost on regular basis. The affected child often lies a lot, initiates fights frequently, is cruel to people, bullies and threatens people of all ages, may engage in gang robbery, or engage in indiscrete precocious sexual activity. The child's behaviour may be so bad that it may bring him or her into conflict with the law. Because of the nature of this disorder, an affected child will usually not benefit from ordinary school life unless specific corrective action is taken early.

Learning Disability

Learning disability is characterised a child's inability to learn within an optimal environment for learning, including an educationally stimulating environment, and adequate provision of resources for the child to learn. Learning disability is thought to be due to the brain's inability to develop optimally, or when the brain has been severely injured at birth or by brain disease in early childhood. The disorder affects approximately 10% of children of school age worldwide.

A child with learning disability may easily lose or misplace items, fail to understand the concept of time in terms of yesterday, today and tomorrow, experience difficulty in understanding and following instructions, have difficulty remembering what he or she might have just been told, and may have trouble mastering reading, spelling, writing, or mathematical concepts and school work. The child may have trouble distinguishing right from left, difficulty identifying words or numbers and may confuse letters of the alphabet or numbers that are mirror images of each other, e.g. 25 and 52, b and d, c and e or p and q. Severe forms of learning disability may be associated with lack of motor coordination, such as inability to walk, hold a pencil or participate in sport.

Learning disability may be mild, moderate, severe or profound in degree, according to the level of social and intellectual impairment that the child suffers. The child with severe or profound learning disability may need total care from others for his or her livelihood and survival. However, a child with mild to moderate learning disability is educable and can be trained to lead simple but successful independent life in later adulthood. A child with mild to moderate learning disability might be found to suffer from specific learning difficulty only, such as reading, writing, or performing arithmetical sums while retaining social skills for other activities required for daily living.

Sleep Disorders in Childhood and Adolescence

Young children may experience severe problems related to their sleep behaviour though these problems rarely reach the health care provider. Five of these disorders include sleep-walking disorder, sleep talking disorder, nightmares and night terror disorder and *pavor nocturnus jactacio.*

Sleep walking disorder

This occurs when the child wakes up in the course of deep sleep and walks and carries out skilful motor activities in the course of walking. Any attempt to wake up the child will fail as the child is typically deeply asleep. At the end of the activity the child will typically return to bed and wake up the following morning without any memory of the events of the previous night.

Sleep talking disorder

This occurs when the child holds a coherent conversation in the course of his or her sleep. Any attempt to interrupt the conversation typically fails as the child is deeply asleep. Sleep talking disorder may co-exist with sleep walking disorder, and the child will typically not remember the conversation the following morning.

Nightmares

These are frightening dreams that seize the child in the course of his or her sleep. The content of the terrifying dream may be related to the experiences of the child earlier in the day. Nightmares occur at a time when the child's sleep is light. As a result the child will vividly recall the content of the dream if waken up, or on the following day. Nightmares are a cardinal feature of the experiences of people who have experienced the traumatic events of armed conflict and war, a horrific accident, or the recurrent bouts of family fights between parents.

Night terror disorder

During *night terror disorder* the child screams in his or her sleep uncontrollably with severe agitation, sweating and with dilated pupils. Any attempt to calm the child up fails as this condition, like sleep walking or talking disorder, occurs when the child is in deep sleep. The episode typically lasts as long as 5-10 minutes and ends spontaneously thereafter when the child returns to sleep.

Pavor nocturnus jactacio

This is a much rarer sleep disorder than the other four. This condition is characterised by the child violently banging his or her head against the bed murmuring and whimpering to him or herself. The child, like in night terror disorder, may be unresponsive to reassurance, and may not recall the

Neurological and neuro-imaging investigations usually yield normal results in parvo nocturnus jactacio and simple cases of sleep walking or sleep talking disorder. However partial seizures, most typically psychomotor epilepsy should be positively ruled out.

HIV/AIDS in Childhood and Adolescence

A child or adolescent may experience the impact of HIV/AIDS in two ways; directly when infected by the AIDS virus, or indirectly when a parent or other significant care-taker falls ill with HIV/AIDS. The child may fall out of school to care for a sick adult, or assume headship of his or her home when the adults die or have to cope with the psychosocial consequences of personally being ill with AIDS. A variety of clinical states have been described in AIDS. Some of these are the result of direct invasion of the brain with the AIDS virus as in dementia related to AIDS, the conversion of the individual's sero-negative health status to sero-positive status, or due to social and personal adjustment problems associated with the awareness that one may be sick with AIDS.

Depression

Depression in childhood related to HIV/AIDS presents with the same clinical features as in other situations and the principles of recognition and diagnosis are the same. Psychological management in this type of depression is usually effective in over 80% of cases. Effectiveness of psychological approach is maximized when the child is helped to verbalize his or her feelings in relation to his or current situation and health. In addition the child or adolescent should be helped to develop strategies to increase his or her ability to respond positively to his or her situation and manage challenges that might threaten his social functioning. Anti-depressant medication is indicated when the depression is severe, associated with suicidal thoughts or is life-threatening in other ways, such as severe psycho-motor retardation.

Anxiety

The child or adolescent with HIV/AIDS might respond to his/ her situation with excessive worrying, experience panic attacks, or show symptoms of phobia or obsessive compulsive disorder. The symptoms of these anxiety disorders are best managed with psychological approaches, which include muscle relaxation exercises, de-conditioning through systematic desensitization, or cognitive behavioural strategies aimed to control obsessions and compulsions.

Seizures

Seizure disorder in HIV/AIDS occurs in some 3% of persons with HIV infection. Seizures are usually the result of extensive involvement of the brain with degeneration, vacuolation or multiple micro-abscesses scattered throughout the brain substance. Convulsions begin late in the course of infection and may present with tonic-clonic convulsions, partial seizures, myoclonus, spasms, or a combination of seizure variants. Prognosis is poor and death painful as the individual usually retains full awareness to the end.

Psychosocial symptoms

Infection with HIV and the development of symptoms of AIDS either in a child, adolescent, or adult care-taker puts a rude end to personal plans and may disorganise the life the child almost irreversibly. The emergence of features of HIV/AIDS may result in shame, guilt feelings, ideas of worthlessness, loss of hope, and loss of interest in planning for the future. Management involves helping the child or adolescent to verbalise his or her feelings, experiences, hopes, plans and strategies he or she might have considered to deal with the situation. Medication is usually not indicated when no evidence of psychiatric disorder is available. Prognosis is usually good and response to psychosocial approaches is excellent.

Effects of Mental disorders in childhood and adolescent

Mental retardation symptoms range from mild, moderate to the severely retarded as follows:-

1. ***Mild retardation:*** usually the symptoms are not easy to detect. There may be slowness in ability to learn. They may go to ordinary schools but may score lowest. They can learn routine tasks and lead fairly independent life.

2. ***Moderately retarded:*** these are easier to note than the first group. They may need to go to special schools where their ability to learn is nurtured differently. They need a lot of things done for them. They are dependant on others than 1st group due to inadequate ability to learn and understand. Their activities may put them to risk as they have poor ability to detect danger. They may commit crimes and may be abused by other people who take advantage of them. Language problems, delayed speech and emotional outbursts are common.

3. ***Severely retarded:*** These children may die early. The few who survive are totally dependant on other people even for feeding, bathing and personal upkeep skills. They cannot sense danger. They may not communicate and play with peers. The condition is usually associated with physical conditions e.g. cerebral palsy, paralysis and deformities.

Management of Mental disorders in childhood and adolescent

1. Manage according to severity through history taking
2. Rule out physical conditions
3. Treat presenting complaints e.g. in restlessness and aggressiveness give haloperidol and phenytoin for fits.
4. Help the child to learn personal care and independence.
5. Work together with parents and help them form support groups to overcome stigma
6. Educate the community on problems and challenges of childhood and adolescence.
7. Refer to special clinics for management of mental problems of children and adolescents.

Management of mental retardation

Depending on the severity:

1. Help the child to learn as much as possible depending on ability to improve personal care and acquire academic knowledge to promote independence.
2. Work together with parents in ensuring the above.
3. Help to initiate support group to overcome stigma.
4. For extreme restlessness and roaming give lower doses of neuroleptic medication, e.g. Haloperidol 2.5 - 5 mgs twice a day.
5. Other problems like fits give Phenytoin 50 - 100 mgs at bedtime.

6. Educate the community on problems and challenges of childhood and adolescence.

Refer to special clinics for management of mental problems.

Helping the Child or Adolescent with Emotional, Psychiatric or Behavioural Problem

- Listen to the child or adolescent and support him or her to express feelings, experiences, and strategies available to cope with the situation.
- Help parents or other adult care-takers to similarly listen to and support the child or adolescent in difficulty.
- Help parents and adult care-takers to exercise tolerance toward difficult adolescent and childhood behaviours.
- Take suicidal or delinquent warnings seriously and develop specific strategies to defuse them early.
- Teach parents to relate to their child or adolescent with emotional, psychiatric or behavioural problems in the same way that they relate to their other children.
- Work with other professions to achieve optimal results, and these other professions include clinical psychologist, social, welfare or probation officer, rehabilitation officer, and the occupational therapist.
- Use appropriate class of medication to control target symptoms.
- Refer difficult childhood or adolescent problems to the specialist early for appropriate assessment, investigations and therapy.

Prevention of Emotional, Mental and Behavioural Problems in Childhood and Adolescence

The prevention of childhood and adolescent emotional, mental and behavioural problems requires a multi-faceted approach involving all concerned with the socialisation process and public health protection. Approaches that need to be considered include the following:

- Adequate nutrition to support optimal growth and development
- Adequate clean water and environmental sanitation
- Protection of the rights and provision of the needs of children and adolescents

- Improved security and protection of communities
- Improved access to democratic systems of governance at all levels
- Promoting universal basic education for all children and adolescents
- Improved access to means of gainful economic livelihood
- Improved reproductive health practice to prevent brain damage
- Early treatment of all childhood febrile conditions, particularly those associated with childhood convulsions in the first five years
- Improved parenting practices
- Early access to medical and or psychosocial support services
- Improved access to psychosocial services for parents with emotional, mental or behavioural problems

28
Enuresis in Childhood and Adolescence

EMILIO OVUGA

Enuresis is the repeated voiding of urine during sleep either by day or at night in bed after reaching the chronological age at which one is expected to have achieved bladder control. Enuresis is diagnosed when an individual passes urine in bed at least twice per week for a period of 3 months after having attained the chronological age at which most people will have achieved bladder control, taken as 5 years of age. Enuresis is a significant condition that interferes with the child's social relations, involvement in social activities such as visiting, and his or her self-confidence and self-esteem.

Classification and etiology

Enuresis is primary if the individual has never achieved bladder control, and secondary if it develops after the individual had achieved bladder control at the expected time. Enuresis tends to run in families. The disorder may be functional when no physical disorder is the cause, and secondary if one can identify a primary physical condition. Physical causes of enuresis include epilepsy, diabetes mellitus and urinary infection. It is important therefore to evaluate every child who presents with enuresis for these disorders before deciding on management measures. If no physical disorder is found, the cause may be psychological such as the birth of a rival sibling, significant family discord between parents, or other stressful social environment in the home of the child. In adults epilepsy is probably the most significant cause of enuresis, followed by diabetes mellitus.

Management of enuresis

Investigate to confirm any physical factor that you suspect at history taking. Provide appropriate physical treatment if physical disorder is confirmed. Provide appropriate psychological treatment if the significant problem is psychosocial in nature. Remember that the child's enuresis may be a symptom of a distressing environment in the home. If this is the case attention should be directed at alleviating the responsible factors at the child's home. If enuresis is purely functional, the treatment of choice is bladder training.

Bladder training technique

Establish baseline information

- Record the number of times the child passes urine during the day.
- Record the number of nights that the child wets his or her bed.
- Record the number of nights when the child does not wet his or her bed.

The enuretic bladder is characteristically sensitive to pressure created by very small quantities of urine. The child with enuresis will pass small quantities of urine several times, up to 7 times per day.

Provide clear instructions

- Take as much water or fluids as you wish between morning and 4.00 o'clock in the evening.
- Do not take any fluid after 4.00 o'clock
- Each time you experience the urge to pass urine, do not rush immediately; hold the urine till you can no longer hold it and then hurry to the toilet.
- Repeat this practice every time you wish to pass urine.
- Record the number of times you pass urine by day time.
- Record the number of nights that you have not passed urine in bed during the week.
- Record the number of nights that you might have passed urine during the week.
- If possible record the volume of urine you pass during the day.
- Record the duration between successive times you pass urine during the day.

Outcome indicators

Explain to the child that if he or she follows the above instructions carefully he or she will note the following measures of his or her success. He or she will:

- Take progressively longer before he gets the urge to pass urine after the last time that he or she passed urine.
- Progressively pass larger volumes every time he or she passes urine.
- Notice fewer nights that he or she passes urine in bed during the week.
- Notice more nights per week that he or she wakes up with a dry bed in the mornings.

Duration of therapy and prognosis

Explain the above procedure and outcome indicators to both the child and mother and ask them to remain patient and optimistic. The role of the mother or other important caretaker will be to provide supervision, moral support, and encouragement to the child without being critical. Highlight the importance of the child recording the parameters listed above, as they will serve as important motivations for the child to achieve the much-needed success that he or she desires.

Explain that it takes two weeks for the child to achieve a cure, but that occasional bed-wetting may occur once or twice in the future. If this happens the child and parent should not get disappointed and the mother should supervise another round of bladder training exercise to boost success.

SECTION IV

Management Approaches in Psychiatry

29
Management of Mental Disorders

EMILIO OVUGA

Introduction

Effective management of mental disorders aims to relieve distress in the affected person and his or her family, and is one of the measures for reducing the rate of mental illnesses in the population. It is also a vehicle for prevention of mental disorders.

Principles of Management of patients with mental disorders

This involves the following:

- Developing a therapeutic relationship with the patients
- Assessment of patient in the course of history taking
- Correct diagnosis of the mental disorder
- Drug treatment
- Use of non-pharmacological forms of treatment e.g. Counselling
- Referral
- Follow up
- Use of support groups
- The compilation of data on mental illness using the Health management information system (HMIS)

A comprehensive assessment of a patient involves the following steps:

- Establish professional relationship (Rapport)
- Obtain patients particulars
- Establish the presenting complaints
- Elicit the history of the presenting complaints
- Establish the past Psychiatric History (including previous treatment).
- Assess the family and social history

- Establish personal history:-
- Birth and early childhood, Schooling, Puberty and adolescent
- Sexual History/behaviour
- Social interaction with others
- Aging (where applicable)
- Occupational history
- Hobbies, leisure and habits
- Marital relationship.
- Carry out physical state assessment

Steps taken in Management of patients with mental disorders

History taking

History taking has two principal functions. It is during the initial stages of history taking that a likely viable therapeutic relationship is established. If the process of history taking is conducted properly, the resulting narrative by the patient of his or her illness experience will promote relief of distress. History taking leads to an understanding of the patient's health problems and the making of the formulation of the patient's problems.

It is on the basis of history taking that useful physical examination, relevant and appropriate bio-psycho-social investigations, and appropriate management programme can be drawn.

- Psychiatric history should be as comprehensive as possible for every patient. Remember that the process of history taking in psychiatry is a continuous process and further clinical encounters with the patient should be used to obtain more information and or to clarify on what is already available.
- Take history not only from the patient but also from significant others where feasible.
- Take detailed history of current psychological illness.
- Take detailed history of current physical health and any previous investigations and treatment received.
- Explore the patient's current and overall life situation.

- Enquire after recent stresses in the life of the patient.
- Identify available social support systems.
- Enquire after family history of similar conditions.

Remember that psychiatric disorders may result from physical illness or present with signs of physical disorder. A particular physical illness episode may be psychological in nature if the following features exist:

- Complaints have been persistent, usually of two years duration.
- The patient has undergone several investigations with negative results.
- The patient has been treated with several medications including herbs with no relief.
- The patient presents with more than four symptoms involving more than two body organ systems.
- Symptom patterns do not follow anatomical patterns.

Very often clues to the possible psychological basis of a patient's health problems can be seen in some of the patient's initial complaints. Important symptoms of psychological disorder include:

- Poor or total lack of sleep. The patient typically wakes up from sleep tired, exhausted and unrefreshed in the mornings.
- Poor or excessive appetite for food.
- General weakness with or without significant weight loss.
- Persistent and unexplained fear for most of the time for at least two weeks.
- Apprehension or the feeling that something tragic is soon going to happen.
- Agitation or the experience of inner tension, unrest, and the inability to relax.
- Persistent and different quality unhappiness for most of the time for at least two weeks.
- Loss of ability to experience pleasure or joy.
- The desire to be alone.

- Irritability over minor distractions or faults by others.
- Difficulty playing useful roles; finding daily work an effort or a burden.
- Difficulty making decisions.
- Difficulty concentrating, absent-mindedness, forgetfulness.
- Too much worrying or thinking.
- Poor relationships with others characterised by complaints of jealousy, envy, and conspiracy to harm or make life difficult.

Clinical assessment

Clinical assessment forms the cornerstone of good psychiatric care. Clinical assessment in psychiatry is primarily concerned with mental status assessment. Mental status may be altered by unrecognised organic factors. Recent or ongoing stressful events may be responsible. Not uncommonly, the "patient" may be a symptom of a troubled family at war with itself. Clinical assessment must therefore be reasonably comprehensive and holistic. However patients are often secretive and may not communicate their health needs readily particularly if they experience suicidal or paranoid feelings, or if their problems stem from troubled family relationships. Clinical assessment of patients/clients includes;

Physical Assessment

a) Treat the patient with respect and tact.

b) Request the patient for permission to be examined. If this is not possible immediately for any reason, ensure that the physical examination is carried out within 24 hours after adequate sedation and control of disturbed behaviour.

c) Look for signs of:

   - Injury, burns, scars, malnutrition, fever, etc.
   - Endocrine, metabolic and haematological disorder.
   - Neurological disease, e.g. muscle wasting, paralysis, deviation of the corner of the mouth of eyes, one-sided bulging of the cheeks, unsteady eyes on gaze to one side, deviation of the tongue to one side, twitches, jerks, inability to sit unaided, unsteady gait, abnormal posture, etc.
   - Structural or functional organ disease, e.g. cardiac valve disease, hypertension, cyanosis, jaundice, rashes and excoriations, etc.

d) Refer to the next higher person in experience in case you are not sure.

Mental Status Assessment

During mental status assessments adequately describe the patient's mental state.

- Avoid the use of technical terms as much as possible unless you are sure of what you want to convey to the reader or yourself.
- Instead, provide excerpts of the mental state with the patient's complaints verbatim where possible.

Mental state comprises of the following elements.

- Appearance.
- Behaviour.
- Speech.
- Thought; namely: delusions and thought progress.
- Perceptions; namely: hallucinations and illusions.
- Cognitive functioning; namely: orientation, concentration, attention span, short-term memory, and long-term memory.
- Insight into health status.

Investigations

There are three principal types of investigation in psychiatry; namely: biomedical investigations, psychological investigations, and social investigations. There are no diagnostic biomedical tests in psychiatry. However when based on careful and comprehensive history, biomedical investigations can save life, and lead to the cure of an organic disorder which might have caused the mental disorder and, lead to significant improvement in patients' quality of life.

Psychological tests (also known as psychometric tests) may be used to confirm a psychiatric diagnosis, decide on the choice of psychotherapy, assess a patient's intelligence or cognitive functioning and assess the prognosis of the patient's illness. Social investigations help in assessing the nature and level of social support available to the patient, and the nature and level of social stressors in the patient's environment; help in the formulation of a patient's health problems; and help in the formulation of an appropriate care programme.

Biomedical Investigations

(i) The type of routine or specialised biomedical investigation to be carried out will usually be determined by findings on history, physical examination, mental status assessment and availability of laboratory facilities at the health unit. When carefully selected the results of well-conducted laboratory tests can aid management immensely.

a) Full haemogram: Hb, ESR, RBC, PCV, MCV, MCHC, Total and differential white cell count, Film comment.
b) Urine analysis: Protein, Sugar, Microscopy, Culture and sensitivity studies.
c) Stool Examination: Ova, Eggs, Cysts, Larvae, and Occult blood.
d) Blood urea and electrolytes.
e) Blood sugar, Glucose tolerance tests.
f) Liver function tests.
g) Widal and Brucella agglutination tests.
h) VDRL, TPHA, HIV screening.
i) CSF studies.
j) TSH, T3, T4, Prolactin level.
k) Urinary 24-hour 17-keto acid assays.
l) Serum lithium level assays.
m) Serum vitamin level assays.
n) Radiological examinations: plain skull x-rays are all that may be conducted at the district hospital level. However more specialised examinations that should be kept in mind, and from which patients may benefit include x-rays with cone view of sella turcica, and electroencephalography, which may be available at the national referral hospital at Mulago hospital, and CT scan. The role of once popular radiological examinations such as carotid angiography, myelography, and pneumoencephalography is probably not certain at this time of development.
o) Electrocardiogram and ultrasound examinations should be available at the regional hospital.

p) Another desirable neurological investigation is MRI which currently is not available in Uganda but might becomeavailable later.

Diagnosis

Diagnosis in psychiatry is dynamic and may change rapidly over time. Some 20% of psychiatric patients in Uganda have multiple diagnoses. Diagnosis forms a firm basis upon which management plans are drawn. For this reason, diagnosis should cover all major aspects of each patient's life. Where a patient is unable to communicate, useful initial data can be obtained from relatives or other persons who might have delivered him/her to the health facility.

Preliminary treatment may then be given based on the information provided. Ensure that you take history and conduct a comprehensive physical and mental state examination within 24 hours of admission. The components of a comprehensive diagnosis should include the following:

Psychiatric disorder

Examples are: Depressive disorder, Anxiety disorder, Delirium.

a) Personality disorder: Examples are: Antisocial personality disorder, Schizoid personality disorder.

b) Physical disorder: Examples are: Hypothyroidism, HIV/AIDS, Neuro-syphilis, Riboflavin deficiency

c) Psychosocial stressor: Examples are Bereavement three months earlier, divorce, loss of employment or social support two weeks prior to onset of illness, Diagnosis of a terminal illness.

d) Level of coping ability: Example are: Inability to do house work, and being confined to bed as a result of illness.

Principles of drug treatment

Drug treatment is just one aspect of psychiatric management. Rapid therapeutic effects are obtained after conducting a careful history and carrying out physical examination and systematic mental status assessment. The use of drugs should not be based on guesswork, but should rely on first principles.

(ii) Make a multi-axial diagnosis (See no. 5 above). Drug treatment for a psychiatric disorder is more likely to yield favourable results if counselling and attention to manipulate stressful events and provide

(iii) Decide what target symptoms you need to control with medication and use specific drugs to control them. For instance:

a) You will need an antidepressant medication if the target symptoms were lack of interest in everything in life; suicidal feelings; and sadness.
b) In case the target symptoms included the patient's belief that he were the president of the whole world and that his enemies were plotting to rob him of the presidency, then you would use a major tranquillizer.

(iv) Decide what the psychiatric disorder is; this makes it possible to choose the appropriate medication. For example:

a) Major Depression is treated with an antidepressant medication
b) Psychosis is treated with a major tranquillizer
c) Panic Disorder is treated with an antianxiety drug
d) Agoraphobia is treated with behavioural psychotherapy and short period of an antianxiety drug
e) Epilepsy that presents with psychological features is treated with an anti-convulsant medication in addition to treating the presenting mental disorder with the appropriate drug such as an anti-depressant, antianxiety medication or a major tranquillizer

(v) Decide what physical condition the patient has in addition to the psychiatric disorder. For instance:

a) AIDS dementia responds suitably to ARV medication
b) Delirium due to vitamin deficiency is treated with B-group of vitamins
c) Delirium to due hypertensive crisis needs an anti-hypertensive drug

(vi) Decide what recent or ongoing psychosocial stressors the patient has experienced.

(vii) Determine the most troubling symptoms.

(viii) Choose the appropriate class of medication to use as indicated above in (iv) and (v) and appropriate dose to start with, based on the patient's age, diagnosis, troubling symptom profile, and severity of condition

(ix) Get familiar with one or two drugs from each class of psychiatric drugs - dosage, route of administration, side-effects, adverse reactions, precautions, contraindications, drug-drug interactions, drug antidotes if any, etc.

(x) Use one drug at a time to reduce side effects, reduce medication-induced functional impairment, and cut costs for patients.

(xi) Avoid combining drugs from the same class of psychotropic medications, e.g chlorpromazine and haloperidol are both major tranquillisers, which act the same way, and there is no advantage in using the two drugs at the same time.

(xii) You may combine drugs from different psychotropic medications if a patient has multiple diagnoses, e.g. depression and schizophrenia.

(xiii) Choose and provide appropriate treatment for any identified physical condition.

(xiv) Decide what strategies to employ in addressing any psychosocial stressors, e.g. you may wish to involve the family, workplace, school, and work with the welfare officer (social worker), the clinical psychologist and the occupational therapist.

(xv) Provide information to the patient and or carer concerning the patient's condition and its management, when recovery or improvement can be expected, treatment side effects, etc.

Involve the patient and or carer in the development of treatment plan including the choice of medications. When in doubt refer to a senior colleague early.

Table 29.2: Basic Information on Psychotropic Drugs Available In Uganda.

Drug	Drug form	Daily dosage range	Route	common side effects	Precautions & contra-Indications
Antidepressant Symptoms: Sadness. Loss of interest. Suicide ideas . Amitryptiline	25 mg Tablets	50-200 mg	Oral	Blurred vision. Dry mouth. Sedation. Increased appetite. Urinary hesitancy. Ejaculatory difficulty. Heat in the body. Psychosis.	Cardiac disease including myocardial infarction & septal defects. Prostate enlargement. Closed angle glaucoma. Liver and renal diseases.
Imipramine	25- Tables	50-200 mg	Oral	Same as for Amitryptiline.	Same as for Amitryptiline.
ANTI-ANXIETY DRUGS Symptoms: Irrational fear Agitation Apprehension Diazepam	5 mg/ml Ampoules	10-20 mg as required	Intravenous or Intramuscularly	Drowsiness. Light-headedness. Ataxia. Dependence.	Pulmonary insufficiency. Respiratory depression. History of dependence.

NEUROLEPTIC DRUGS Symptoms: Hallucinations Delusions Irrational behaviour Chlorpromazine	25,50, 100 mg Tablets. 50 mg Ampoules	100-1000 mg	Oral or Intra-muscular injection.	Parkinsonism. Dystonia. Akathisia. Akinesia. Hypothermia. Hyperpyrexia.	Coma due to central nervous system depression. Liver disease.
Haloperidol	5, 10 mg Tablets. 5, 50, 100 mg Ampoules.	5-80 mg daily or 50-150 mg every 4 weeks.	Oral or by deep intra-muscular.	As for chlorpromazine.	As for chlorpromazine.
Trifluoperazine	2, 5, 10, 15 mg	2-60 mg	Oral	As for chlorpromazine	As for chlorpromazine
Thioridazine	25, 50, 100 mg Tablets.	150-800 mg	Oral	As for chlorpromazine Pigmentation of retina with impaired night vision.	Regular eye check in long-term use.

ANTI-MANIC DRUGS Symptoms: Elated mood Irritable mood Grandiose delusions Increased sociability Lithium carbonate	250, 300, 400, 500 mg Tablets.	250-1000 mg	Oral	Gastro-intestinal disturbance. Poly-uria. Polydypsia. Fine tremors. Dizziness. Ataxia. Muscle weakness. Drowsiness.	Check renal, thyroid function. Full haemogram. Monitor renal and thyroid function. Check serum thyroid hormoe levels every three months. Serum level should not exceed 1.2 mM/l.

Table 29.2: continued

Drug	Drug form	Daily dose	Route	Side effects	Precautions & contra-indications
Anticonvulsants Carbamazepine	100, 200 mg Tablets; 100 mg/5ml liquid.	100-1200 mg	Oral	Gastro-intestinal Disturbance. Dizziness. Drowsiness Ataxia. Confusion. Agitation. Convulsions. Skin rashes within2-4 weeks. Exfoliative dermatitis.	Discontinue use if rashes, confusion, convulsions develop within 2-4 weeks.
Phenytoin	50, 100 mg tablets or capsules	100-300 mg	Oral	Gum swelling, Poor oral hygiene. Peripheral neuropathy. Ataxia. Anaemia. Skin rashes. Headache. Confusion.	Discontinue or reduce dose if side effects persist.
Ethosuximide	250 mg capsules. 250 mg/5ml syrup.	250 mg/day for children up to 6 Years. 250-500 mg/day for children older than 6 years. 500-1500 mg/day in adults.	Oral	Gastrointestinal disturbance. Drowsiness. Dizziness. Ataxia. Photophobia. Leucopoenia and agranulocytosis are rare.	Renal and liver disease. Pregnancy. Breast feeding.

Sodium Valproate	200 mg tablets	200-600 mg/day.	Oral	Nausea. Ataxia. Skin rashes. Tremors. Bleeding. Liver impairment.	Do not withdraw suddenly.
Anti-parkinsonian drug Benzhexol	2 mg tablets	2-15 mg/day. Use only when the patient develops extra-pyramidal symptoms on Neuroleptic.	Oral	Mental confusion. Dry mouth. Paralytic ileum. Dizziness. Blurred vision.	Cardiovascular, liver or renal Impairment. Liable to be abused. Avoid sudden Withdrawal and routine use.

Rapid Neuroleptisation

This term refers to the administration of relatively high potency anti-psychotic medication in sufficient frequency to achieve rapid control of psychotic symptoms within the shortest time. This method of drug management is recommended only for use by psychiatrists, but is described here to show the feasibility of rapid control of distressing behaviour and experience caused by mental illness. Appropriate referral is advised if control is not achieved within 24 hours.

The objective of rapid Neuroleptisation is to achieve rapid control of psychotic disruptive assaultive and dangerous behaviour. The specific objectives of rapid Neuroleptisation are three-fold, namely:

- To avoid patient distress.
- To protect the patient and other people from potential injury.
- To avoid or shorten the duration of possible hospitalisation

An expeditiously carried out rapid Neuroleptisation is desirable for the following reasons, namely:

- The calm and order created at home or on a hospital ward.
- A boost to staff morale.
- Reduction in burn-out.
- Reduction in the amount of possible litigation.

Symptom Profile

Rapid Neuroleptisation may be indicated if the following constellation of symptoms is observed: agitation, destructiveness, hostility, assaultive behaviour, pressure of speech, incoherent thought and speech, delusions and hallucinations.

Diagnostic Profile

The patient who requires rapid Neuroleptisation would most likely have any of the following diagnoses.

- Acute schizophrenia with excitement or marked withdrawal.
- Acute mania with excitement.
- Delirium.
- Delirium tremens.

Pre-treatment Work-up

Before the course of treatment is commenced, ensure that a thorough physical work-up is carried and special attention should be paid to the following:

- Cardiovascular status - hypertension, hypotension, arrhythmias.
- Possibility of head injury.
- Signs of space occupying lesions and focal neurological signs.
- Epilepsy.
- Diabetes mellitus.
- Electrolyte imbalance.
- Anti-cholinergic intoxication - the known psychiatric patient.

It is necessary that rapid Neuroleptisation is supported by:

- An accurate diagnosis.
- Identified symptoms that respond to neuroleptic medication.
- Evidence of a comprehensive physical examination.

If physical examination cannot be carried out immediately due to the level of agitation, etc, this should be documented and an initial low neuroleptic dose should be used combined with 10-20 mg of diazepam intravenously to achieve sedation. An attempt should then be made to carry out some physical examination to determine vital physiological signs before Neuroleptisation can be commenced.

Drugs and Administration

Injection Sites

One of two principal injection sites may be used, namely: the deltoid muscle and the gluteus maximus muscle. Of these two, the deltoid muscle is better as absorption from this site is faster than from the gluteal region. If the latter site is chosen, the upper outer quadrant region should be used to avoid injury to the sciatic nerve.

Under no circumstances should a neuroleptic drug be administered intravenously unless the manufacturer's enclosed leaflet indicates so. Even then the drug concerned should be administered slowly to avoid thrombophlebosis (inflammation, swelling and pain) in the affected arm.

The drug of choice for rapid Neuroleptisation is Haloperidol. In its absence chlorpromazine may be used.

Haloperidol:

1. Begin with an initial dose of 10-15 mg I.M.I.
2. Thereafter administer the drug in doses of 2-10 mg every 30 - 60 minutes till a total dose of 60 mg in 24 hours has been achieved or psychotic symptoms have been brought under effective control.

Chlorpromazine:

1. Begin with an initial dose of 100 mg I.M.I.
2. Thereafter administer the drug in doses of 50 - 100 mg every 30 - 60 minutes until a total dose of 700 - 800 mg in 24 hours has been achieved or psychotic symptoms have been effectively controlled.

After the control of psychotic behaviour and symptoms has been achieved, oral medication can safely be started six to eight hours after the last dose of injection. The dose required for oral medication should preferably be double that used in rapid Neuroleptisation procedure.

Precautions

The following precautions should be taken while the patient is under-going rapid Neuroleptisation, namely: monitor vital physiological signs every 30 minutes to two hours depending on the dose of neuroleptic used and the general physical health of the patient. Should signs of autonomic instability be noticed, an intravenous fluid therapy should be started and the process of rapid Neuroleptisation should be stopped immediately and the more conventional, less intensive method of medication should be used.

Expected Outcomes

Effective rapid Neuroleptisation should lead to the patient being calm and cooperative with no signs of agitation or anxiety in less than 24 hours.

Side-effects

Expected side effects to rapid Neuroleptisation are the usual ones encountered neuroleptic medication, namely: Parkinsonism, akinesia, akathisia, acute dystonic reactions, laryngeal or pharyngeal dystonia, severe hypotension, cardiac arrhythmias and or cardiac arrest, catatonia, and the malignant neuroleptic syndrome. To avoid the distress associated with these side effects, an "as necessary dose of benzhexol prescription" should be provided for the nurses to administer if they occur. Cardiac arrhythmias and arrest are extremely rare. Malignant neuroleptic syndrome is potentially fatal and the offending medication should be discontinued immediately once the problem is detected. Immediate life support measures consisting of intra-venous fluid therapy, anti-pyretic medication, and investigations to exclude a physical condition for the fever should be instituted. In addition, a consultation to the physician should be urgently sent.

30
Drugs Used in Psychiatry

EMILIO OVUGA

Introduction

Drugs that are used in the treatment of mental disorders are called psychotropic drugs, meaning affecting the mind (Cookson, Taylor and Katona, 2002). Psychotropic drugs are classified according to their main clinical effects on mental disorder. The use of these drugs is largely determined by the presence of what are known as target symptoms, which also form part of the main symptoms required to make a diagnosis of respective mental disorder. Table 1 below depicts the classification of drugs in common use in Uganda. (See Table 1)

Antidepressants

Antidepressants are used in the treatment of major depression. On the average Tricyclic antidepressants begin to show clinical effect after 10-14 days of daily use. The evidence that they are working is shown by the reduction of experience of sadness, improvement in the level of interest and the loss of suicidal feelings if these have been reported by the patient at initial or review interviews. Some antidepressants, particularly of the SSRI group may also be used in the treatment of phobias, obsessive-compulsive disorder and panic disorder.

Antipsychotics

Antipsychotics are also known as neuroleptics. The term neuroleptic was attached to this group of drugs because they work by acting on brain cells (neurons); neuroleptic literally means seizes the brain. Evidence of clinical effect comprises of reduction of excited violent noisy behaviour that is replaced by quietude (apathy), lessening of hallucinations and gradual loss of delusions and other symptoms associated with these.

Table 30. 1: Classification of drugs used in psychiatry

Class of drug	Sub-class	Examples	Mental disorder	Target symptom	Comments
Antidepressants	Tricyclic antidepressants	Imipramine Amitriptyline	Major depression	Sadness, loss of interest, suicide behaviour	On the essential drugs list
	SSRIs	Fluoxetine Paroxetine Sertraline	Major depression	Sadness, loss of interest, suicide behaviour	Available on the open market
Neuroleptics	Pheno-thiazines	Chlorpromazine Thioridazine Trifluoperazine Fluphenazine	Psychotic disorders	Hallucinations, delusions, irrational behaviour	On the essential drugs list
	Butyro-phenones	Haloperidol	Manic disorder	Elated mood, expansive self-image, grandiose delusions	On the essential drugs list
	Thio-xantines	Flupentixol	Psychotic disorder	Hallucinations, delusions	Available on the open market
Atypical anti-psycho tics		Risperidone Clozapine Olanzapine	Psychotic disorder	Hallucinations, delusions	Available on the open market

Anti-anxiety drugs	Benzo-diazepines	Diazepam	Anxiety disorder	Irrational fear Agitation Apprehension	On the essential drugs list
Mood stabilizers	Lithium	Lithium carbonate	Manic depressive psychosis	Manic symptoms alternate with symptoms of depression	On the essential drugs list
	Anti-convulsants	Carbamazepine Valproate	Manic depressive psychosis	Manic symptoms alternate with symptoms of depression	On the essential drugs list
	Atypical antipsycho-tics	Clozapine Risperidone Olanzapine	Recurrent episodes of manic depressive psychosis	Recurrent episodes disrupt normal life of the client	Available on the open market

Antianxiety drugs (Anxiolytic drugs)

This group of drugs is used in the treatment of anxiety disorders. Diazepam is often used along with an antipsychotic to achieve rapid control of symptoms in the excited patient. Diazepam or Chlordiazepoxide are also use in the detoxification of alcohol withdrawal states and the treatment of sleep disorder such as insomnia. These drugs have a high potential to cause dependence and should not be used in excess of 10-14 days.

Mood stabilisers

These drugs are used in the treatment of manic illness and in the prevention of relapses of manic episodes. Their use in the prevention of relapses may be indicated by the occurrence of at least three episodes within 12 months while the client has been using an antipsychotic drug.

Side Effects

Drugs used in psychiatry often cause unpleasant side-effects that include sedation, mental dullness, problems with movement coordination and dry mouth. The drugs that are not on the essential drugs list produce less side-effect, work faster and promote overall quality of life better than the conventional drugs that are available on the official list, but are costly. To minimize the experience of side-effects and to help the client contain the cost of medication in the event that he/she has to purchase drugs from the open market it might be useful:

- Not to use more than two drugs unless indicated; when in doubt consult or refer the client to a senior colleague
- Not to combine the use of two drugs from the same class, e.g. Haloperidol and chlorpromazine or Imipramine and Amitryptiline
- To explain the potential side-effects the client is likely to experience
- To indicate how long it will take before acute symptoms will disappear, and for how long the use of drugs will continue thereafter
- To explain what potential dangers might arise consequent upon the use of psychotropic drugs and how the dangers might be prevented
- To keep drugs out of the rich of children
- To consult or refer to a senior colleague if a child requires psychotropic drug

31
Management of Excited Behaviour

EMILIO OVUGA

Violence and excited behaviour constitute a psychiatric emergency. Violence, excitement, disturbed behaviour is one of the commonest reasons that necessitate admission to hospital. The rapid control of violence and excitement should therefore be one of the top priorities in the care of the patient in order that the patient is relieved of his/her distress without much delay.

The rapid control of violence and or excited behaviour restores order and lost dignity to the patient and his or her family. In addition the successful and speedy control of symptoms is likely to send the correct message to the community that the control and treatment of mental illness by western medicines is feasible.

This module provides skills and knowledge on various methods the participants can immediately apply to control symptoms so as to help the mentally ill client to work and social network, and prevent the disruption of social set up.

The new patient who is excited or excitable

- Invite the patient to sit down with you for discussion if this is possible.
- Ask relatives or the police to remove mechanical restraints after having obtained the patient's willingness to be non-violent.

General measures in the control of excited behaviour

- Sit face-to-face with the patient and speak to him/her directly, gently and clearly so that you can be understood without ambiguity.
- Ensure that arrangements for your personal security are in place; do not sit in such a position as to be easily trapped.
- Always have arrangements for the emergency drug control of violent behaviour made ready.
- In the case of violent behaviour all staff must act together and should desist from being played against each *other by patients.*

- Use reasonable physical restraint to facilitate drug administration as indicated.
- Ensure that you actively exclude any physical cause for the violent behaviour and provide appropriate treatment.
- Nurse the violent and excited patient in exclusion in a quiet room only for the minimum necessary period.
- Monitor physiological signs every 2-4 hours in the first 12 hours and then daily thereafter until the patient's situation improves.
- Involve other team members in the care of the patient.
- Refer the patient to other professional colleagues early if the situation so demands.

Attend to the general needs of the patient while under heavy sedation. These needs include:

- Fluids by mouth or intravenously.
- Adequate aeration of the seclusion room.
- Access to proper excreta disposal facilities.
- Monitor vital physiological functions, temperature, blood pressure, pulse rate.

Establish measures to prevent patient harming him/her-self. These include:

- Padded room.
- No rails to hang from.
- No items to use for hanging self.
- Regularly monitor the patient.

As soon as violence is under control take full history about the patient's whole mental health problems. Institute appropriate management programme.

Communication guidelines in the control of excited behaviour

- Do not challenge the patient or argue with him/her.
- Remember that any undesirable behaviour needs to be understood and appropriately addressed therapeutically.

- Reassure the patient that you have no intentions to harm him/her but rather help him or her.
- Encourage the patient to explain to you the origins and basis of his/her situation.
- Document the salient features of the violent behaviour with the permission of the patient as the narrative proceeds.
- Let the patient know that you have understood the problem through clarifying comments and questions.
- Propose and explain a course of treatment and other care options and request the patient to agree to their implementation.
- Administer effective doses of neuroleptic drugs.

Drug Management in case of excited behaviour

- Use at least the minimum equivalent dose of 200-300 mg of chlorpromazine as a start dose for the healthy adult patient. (See table 3).
- Repeat the dose of the chosen drug in the equivalent dose of 200 mg chlorpromazine every 8 hours for the next 2-3 doses intra-muscularly.
- The last dose of intra-muscular dose of medication must be followed immediately eight hours later with the equivalent of 200-300 mg of chlorpromazine and maintained every 8 hours until symptom control. This may take 2-3 weeks to achieve. (Also refer to section on rapid Neuroleptisation below).
- Following the adequate control of violence or excitement, the dose of medication may be reduced in the equivalent of 100 mg chlorpromazine every 1-2 weeks.

The hospitalised patient who is excitable or excited

Excitement with or without violence on a hospital ward can usually be predicted and prevented. Such behaviour may be due to the boring routines on the ward and or poor control of mental disorders commonly associated with violent aggressive manipulative behaviour in some patients. The early recognition and prevention of violence can be achieved by being alert to the possible occurrence of such behaviour. The patient who is likely to be violent has the following features.

- Complains against staff and patients and threatens assault.
- Withdraws from others.
- Lacks sleep and appetite.
- Clinical behaviour pattern fluctuates.
- Refuses medication.

Management of excited behaviour

1. Attend to potential violent behaviour at the earliest sign.
2. Enter into a contract and develop a set of strategies with the individual concerned to address the problem in question.
3. Seclude the individual when necessary.
4. Review the physical and mental health of the person.
5. Change medication as necessary.

Home Care

It is not advisable to provide care for the violent noisy patient at home. However, relatives may wish to supervise medication at home on outpatient basis. Under such circumstances a decision to provide treatment on outpatient basis may be based on the overall severity and other aspects of the clinical problem. The outcome of home care supervised by relatives is usually quite good and may be encouraged.

1. Conduct a full psychiatric history, physical examination and mental state examination.
2. Explain the nature of clinical problem in simple language, repeating if necessary, before the patient and relatives leave for home.
3. Explain the treatment plan and ensure that the patient and relatives understand what to do at home.
4. Explain all potential side effects of medication supplied.
5. Supply medication for 3-7 days at a time.
6. Explain the likely clinical outcome on medication, indicating particularly when control of symptoms is expected.

7. Give an appointment for the patient and relatives to come for review every 3-7 days.

8. Instruct the relatives and patient to contact you in the meantime or come for the review earlier as necessary.

9. Warn relatives of potential suicide behaviour particularly if the clinical diagnosis is depressive disorder and or evidence of suicide behaviour has been detected in the course of assessment.

10. Use the same drug doses as recommended above. For less severe problems lower doses may be used eight hourly orally.

Table 31.1: Current dose equivalents of available psychiatric drugs to 200-300 mg of chlorpromazine

Drug	Dose	Frequency	Route
Haloperidol injection	15-20 mg	Start	I.M.I
Haloperidol Tablet	15-20 mg	8 hourly	Oral
Trifluoperazine Tablet	15-20 mg	8 hourly	Oral

32

If a Patient is not Improving Adequately

EMILIO OVUGA

If a patient shows no satisfactory improvement

- Assess the patient for signs of expected side effects of medication, e.g. dry mouth, tremors, rigidity, rabbit posturing.
- Estimate serum drug level to compare with recommended therapeutic level if there are facilities for doing so.
- Estimate serum Prolactin level if it is feasible to do so. For instance the optimal serum level for adequate control of psychotic symptoms on neuroleptic medication is 16-30 ng/ml
- Re-assess the diagnosis by reviewing history, physical and mental status assessment.
- Carry out relevant laboratory investigations.
- Increase or lower the dose of medication as required.
- Consider change of medication to a different class of psychiatric drugs.
- Eliminate offending medication if judged responsible for lack of improvement.
- Discuss the clinical problem with colleagues if any.
- Consult physician or other specialist as indicated or transfer to a better equipped health unit.
- Re-assess the patient's social circumstances if not yet done.
- Carry out psychological assessment, personality test, and intelligence test.
- Attend to general fluid and electrolyte balance.
- Ensure that the patient and carer understand the nature of the patient's clinical situation. Go over instructions, clarifications, and explanations required to enhance quick recovery.

33
Compliance

EMILIO OVUGA

Compliance refers to the adherence of the patient to medical advice, follow treatment instructions, and change his/her behaviour in order to enhance recovery from an illness episode, maintain good health and promote personal health. Poor compliance refers to the patient's failure to follow medical advice. Several reasons explain poor compliance, namely:

- Socio-cultural factors such as knowledge, attitudes, beliefs and practices: a person who believes his/her condition to be due to cultural or home problems might not adhere to medical advice
- Fear of loss of personal control
- Fear of stigmatisation
- Drug side effects and adverse reactions
- Lay beliefs regarding cure; a drug that achieves quick relief of symptoms will be discontinued before the full clinical recovery from illness episode
- Adverse social circumstances
- Lack of social support system
- Poverty
- A long distance to health facility to collect medication or attend reviews may lead to non-adherence to medical advice
- Lack of trust and respect for the health care provider may lead to the drug that he/she has prescribed not being used

The relationship between insight and compliance is complex. Compliance is good when insight is lacking but may become poor when insight returns, especially among individuals with manic or paranoid disorders. In general insight is good when an individual has attained full recovery, particularly after counselling and provision of information.

Poor compliance is undesirable because it leads to a vicious cycle of poor health, poor functional ability, and poor economic power, worsening of social circumstances, and deteriorating interpersonal relationships. Promoting compliance is thus an essential task in the care of the mentally sick.

1. Treat the patient politely and with due respect.
2. Provide clear information to the patient and carers about his/her condition, i.e. illness causes, aggravating factors, prevention, course and prognosis.
3. Provide information on the type of treatment, treatment outcome, treatment side effects and possible adverse reactions. Provide information on the prevention of expected side effects and adverse reactions.
4. Avoid challenging the patient or arguing with him/her over his/her views, delusions, beliefs, hallucinations and life problems. Remember that the illness experiences of the patients are real and warrant empathy, sympathy and due understanding.
5. Teach the patient and carer about the early warning signs of illness relapse.
6. Encourage the patient to express his/her feelings, ideas, experiences, fantasies, fears, and real life problems.
7. Identify harmful behavioural patterns and talk them through with the patient and carer.
8. Respect the right of the patient and carer to consult traditional healer while encouraging the need to follow medical advice.
9. Involve social support system in care, clinical supervision and the supervision of medication.
10. Identify and address adverse social circumstances.
11. Determine the functional capacity of the patient and plan rehabilitation with the patient and carer accordingly.
12. Discuss the economic problems affecting the patient and help the patient with possible strategies to solve them.

13. Support the patient and carer through counselling to help them cope with illness and identified life problems.

14. Take drug side-effects seriously.

Compliance is likely to improve if you can identify the most troubling symptoms, their causes and their negative impact on the patient and other people in his/her social milieu from the perspective of the patient and use these to justify the need for the patient to follow medical advice. In addition you might wish to talk about your experience in providing care to other patients with similar problems and how those patients improved their compliance abilities.

N.B Drugs used in mental health do cause unpleasant side effects, which may need to be taken seriously to show the patient that you too are concerned about their effect on the person concerned; the side-effects include: protruding tongue, excessive salivation, eyes rolling upwards, tremors of the hands, drowsiness, weight gain, shuffling gait and neck stiffness.

34
Non-pharmacological Methods of Treatment in Psychiatry

EMILIO OVUGA

Effective treatment of persons with mental illness is not only by use of drugs but also by the use of non-pharmacological methods and common ones include: -

1. **Counselling:** This is the process of talking with a person with problems with a view to provide supportive encouragement, guidance and understanding to help the individual cope, manage and or live with his or her problems.

2. **Psychotherapy:** This is the process of discussing with or enabling the person with problems in such way as to help the individual express their emotions and eventually get better e.g. cognitive therapy.

3. **Occupational therapy:** This is the process of engaging the patient in appropriate activities to occupy the patient's mind, reactivate the previous skills or acquire new ones as part of treatment.

4. **Recreation therapy:** This is the process of engaging the patient in social activity like listening to music, participating football, drama and dance as a means of processing personal problems and channeling them through meaningful avenues in order to attain relief, etc.

5. **Support groups:** These are advocacy groups; composed of patients, care takers/relatives and other concerned members of the community e.g. Schizophrenic Fellowship, Alcoholic Anonymous, Mental Health Uganda and Epilepsy support Association.

Health workers are encouraged to mobilise and sensitize the community about the importance of formation of support groups to promote mental health, reduce relapses, promote healthy lifestyles and sustain good health overall.

35
Psychological Impact of Trauma

EMILIO OVUGA

Introduction

The psychological outcomes of the experience of trauma are so real that it may be difficult even for victims themselves to believe in them. Yet disasters, whether natural as in the form of a house collapsing or man-made as in the case of repeated domestic violence and genocide are common place. This chapter outlines key issues about the psychological consequences of trauma also known as post-traumatic stress disorder (PTSD).

Definition

PTSD is mental disorder that follows the experience of severe trauma that is beyond the tolerance of the ordinary human being.

Prevalence

The exact figure of how common PTSD is remains difficult to establish. What is clear is that soon after the occurrence of trauma affecting whole communities the prevalence of symptoms of PTSD can be detected among 80-90%. However as time elapses, this prevalence will drop considerably over the next six months to about a third of the population, and this figure will continue to drop over the next year or so to less than 10%.

Causes

The causes of PTSD may be categorised into two broad groups as depicted in table 1 below.

Table 35.1: Causes of post-traumatic stress disorder

Natural disaster	Man made disaster
Storm	Domestic violence
Floods	Rape and defilement

Natural disaster	Man made disaster
Bush fire	Armed conflict
Earthquake	War
Bus or other accident	Political terror
	Suicide bombing
	Hostage taking

The causes of PTSD vary as is shown in the summary in table 1 and they range from rape, child abuse, and domestic violence to armed conflict and war, suicide bombing or political terror meted out on the populace by their own governments as an instrument of domination (Herman, 1992). The common factor in these varied causes of trauma is the intense feeling of danger, the imminent threat of death and personal annihilation, the loss of control, and the intense feeling of helplessness.

Trauma may be experienced directly by the victim, perpetrator, rescue team members and media personnel or indirectly by other people through witnessing when one is present at the time of the occurrence of the trauma, report made by witnesses, viewing the events of the trauma on television, reading about the trauma or seeing the photographs of trauma events and victims.

Who is liable to suffer from PTSD?

PTSD may affect literally every one who is exposed to the events of trauma. These include both the perpetrator of the trauma and the victim directly or indirectly as well as bystanders or other people who witness, are informed, who view or read about the events of trauma in the print or electronic media.

Painful experiences in trauma

People who are trapped in trauma situations experience

- Terror – intense fear that eventually fades away to leave the victim feeling helpless
- Disconnection – the individual feels cut-off, separated from family and friends; he/she becomes isolated

- Captivity – the individual feels trapped, prisoner, in the full control of the trauma situation; he/she depends on the trauma situation or on fate for his/her personal safety and survival
- Sense of abandonment; loss of trust – in the hour of need the individual lacks access to sources of any help and support

Issues in trauma experience

Though the painful occurrence of trauma is common, society and individual members of the society often advocate for victims to remain silent, adhere to the unspoken oath of secrecy and to deny the reality of the trauma at all costs. This is expected as to admit the experience of trauma may be seen as a sign of moral weakness, and may attract guilt feelings and self-blame for exposing oneself to the events of trauma; society often blames victims for their part in the events of the trauma.

Manifestations of trauma experience

Many victims learn to cope with their trauma experiences in the community partly with support from their communities and partly learning to live with the aftermath of trauma experience. Those individuals who fail to cope with symptoms of PTSD may use alcohol excessively for self-medication against anxiety, depression and early severe mental illness and to induce sleep, or engage in suicide behaviour. Children cope with their trauma experience by replaying the events of trauma that they might have witnessed or experienced. For example it has been common for children from northern Uganda to re-enact the horrifying events of raids by the Lord's Resistance Army during play times.

Symptoms and signs of PTSD

- Disbelief; unwillingness to accept that the events of trauma have occurred.
- Emotional numbness; being unable to feel sad or joyful
- Impaired capacity for human relations; being unable to form warm trusting relations with other persons, particularly members of the opposite sex as occurs after rape.
- Sleep disturbance; poor or total lack of sleep due to frightening dreams about the events of trauma.
- Loss of appetite for food

- Flashbacks; experiencing the events of trauma in full wakefulness, e.g. hearing victims crying and pleading for mercy like flash of lightning.
- Hallucinations; experiencing the events of trauma in great detail in full wakefulness, e.g. the act of torturing and killing a victim.
- Re-experience of trauma in situations that serve as reminders of trauma, e.g. every time people who have been abducted by the Lord's Resistance Army pass by where they were abducted they re-experience the full events of the abduction.
- Avoidance of situations that remind the victim of the trauma.
- Irritability; getting upset easily.
- Unpredictable episodes of aggression and violence.
- Increased fear reaction; being jumpy at every sound, being ready to flee.
- Depression, anxiety, alcohol abuse, suicide behaviour.
- More complicated signs:
    - An individual acts under another personality, as if there are more individuals in one body.
    - An individual's behaviour changes unpredictably from warm friendly to being upset, violent.
    - An individual loses function of part of the body, e.g. being blind, deaf or paralysed when he/she is not.
    - Having numerous symptoms, such as body pains and aches that do not respond to medication.

Complications of PTSD

Common complications in PTSD include:
- Alcohol abuse
- Suicide behaviour
- Chronic depression
- Anxiety disorder

Helping people with trauma

Helping people with trauma in primary care requires that one can recognise them in the first place, and this may not be easy. A useful tip to remember

Uganda is a traumatized society and people with trauma may be common in primary care.

Useful clues to the recognition of the individual with the effects of trauma are:

- Multiple body pains and aches
- Problem of alcohol or other drug abuse
- Vague general symptoms
- Individual comes from current or previous war zone
- Individual is a child or young adult of both sexes

The psychological approach to helping is perhaps the best approach to care as this method will help the individual achieve reconnection to other caring human beings, regain lost control and autonomy, regain lost trust and confidence, achieve a validation of his/her experiences and escape from captivity through talk therapy. To help the individual achieve these goals the following five questions in talk therapy may be asked over a course of 4 to 6 sessions:

1. How has the experience of trauma affected your life personally? (e.g. change in the person of the individual, behaviour patterns, feelings, thoughts)
2. What are the main problems that you have experienced often or repeatedly as a result of the trauma? (e.g. threats to occupation, human relations)
3. How have you coped with the problems that you have mentioned or talked about? (e.g. what has he/she done about personal experiences? Does he/she use prayers, isolate self, use alcohol, or feel suicidal?)
4. How else could you deal with these problems? (e.g. what alternative ways are available for getting over the effects of the trauma? who are there to confide in?)
5. How do you plan to reconstruct your life from now on? (e.g. What plans are available for the future to get over the trauma and move on?)

Appropriate medication to treat depression, anxiety or other forms of mental disorder may be used if indicated. Very often the need for medication will recede as the individual improves on talk therapy. When in doubt refer to a senior early

36
Traditional Medicine

CATHERINE ABBO

Introduction

Over 80% of the population in developing countries goes to traditional healers for their health problems; 40% of these do so for mental health problems (Abbo, 2004). Traditional medicine is also known as complementary or alternative medicine. Traditional healing practices include a wide range of practical health approaches, knowledge and beliefs that incorporate the use of plant and animal products, mineral-based medicines, spiritual treatments and manual techniques that aim to achieve and maintain the wellbeing of individuals as well as to prevent the occurrence of illness.

Definitions

A traditional healer is a person who is recognised by the community in which he/she lives as someone who is able and skilled to provide health care by using plant and/or animal products and mineral substances or other methods based on social, cultural and religious background, and on the knowledge, attitudes and beliefs that are prevalent in the community regarding physical, mental and social wellbeing as well as illness and disability.

A witchdoctor is a person who ascertains the cause of illness or misfortune by the use of divine or magical powers. Witchcraft is the practice of determining the cause illness or other misfortune by the use of magical powers or sorcery.

The term witchcraft is reserved for the use of magical powers for evil purposes (charm). Traditional medicine is often used to reduce the power of witchcraft, or treat and make harmless the supposed effect of the witchcraft. Witchcraft is not the same as traditional medicine and the two should not be confused.

Beliefs about witchcraft and evil spirits

People often feel that witchcraft or evil spirits have caused their illness, or that supernatural forces are responsible for their condition. Avoid challenging beliefs as these as opposing such beliefs might make the person feel uncomfortable about discussing their illness and coping mechanisms freely with the health care provider. Instead it might be useful to encourage the individual to disclose his/her belief systems about the cause of his/her illness, and understand them from the patient's view point before offering an alternative medical explanation in simple terms.

Categories of traditional healers

Three broad categories of traditional healers exist, though there is often no sharp distinction between them. Many healers use a combination of healing procedures.

Herbalists

These are healers who use plants and their roots or animal products. The products are typically applied through scarification, steam baths, or mixed with mineral substances.

Diviners (Spiritualists)

This group of healers consults spirits to identify the type and cause of illness. Diviners often differentiate between normal health problems such as cancer, diabetes mellitus or AIDS, and traditional health problems that involve the control or removal of evil spirits.

Faith healers

These are healers who recite verses from the Quran or the Holy Bible to achieve healing.

Training of traditional healers

Approximately 80% of traditional healers suffered from some form of mental health problem before becoming healers (Ovuga, Boardman and Oluka, 2001). This usually follows the person being identified and trained by an attending practicing traditional healer at the healer's shrine. Other healers report having been called to the profession in dreams during sleep and some become healers by inheritance and apprenticeship within the family.

Factors that influence the choice of health care

Various factors influence the use of traditional healers' services often in combination with the use of hospital services.

- **Community perception:** The community believes that some conditions are caused by cultural and traditional problems and are therefore not treatable using modern western medicines. This belief often makes the service user to consciously decide which health care to use though at great cost sometimes. Remember though that most people who seek traditional health care or cultural and religious services for such reasons as to prevent death or ill-health, end misfortunes, bring about good luck, become rich, or secure the love of someone have significant mental health problems.
- **Accessibility:** The services of traditional healers are often accessible, readily available, affordable, flexible and appropriate to the cultural setting. Traditional healers share the same concepts of disease and misfortunes as their communities.
- **Dissatisfaction:** Frequently cited inadequacies in drug supplies, the attitudes of health care providers and the distance to health units often discourage people from using modern health facilities.
- **Combined use:** Evidence shows that communities use both modern health facilities and traditional healers' shrines for health care. It is possible that the two groups of health care providers might contribute to community health if there was a system of communication exchange between them.
- **Holistic approach:** It is now recognised that the combined efforts of modern health care providers and traditional healers can work to calm patients and facilitate healing through the elimination of stress that might result from unfamiliar treatment procedures. A patient who has faith in the healing powers of traditional medicine can derive from it a sense of acceptance, belonging and awareness of self in the midst of fear, suffering and death; this helps to alleviate pain and distress by facilitating the healing process.

The role of traditional healers

Traditional healers are useful in primary health care for the following reasons. The healers:

- Treat common mental disorders in the community
- Conduct Counselling (talk therapy) around the health problems that their patients bring to them
- Treat psychosocial problems such as problems within the family.

Walking together with traditional healers

Formation of liaison services with traditional healers at primary health care level might improve mental health service delivery and the quality of mental health care. Traditional healers could be active case finders and their involvement might facilitate early referrals, monitoring and follow-up. With adequate training traditional healers could help in educating the community and in helping to demystify the management of psychiatric disorder, destigmatise mental illness and those who suffer from mental disorder, and to destigmatise mental illness. Traditional healers are good mobilisers by virtue of the respect they command in their communities and their involvement could easily contribute to the success of mental health programs in a decentralised district health care system.

SECTION V

Miscellaneous

37
The Mental Treatment Act

EMILIO OVUGA

Introduction

Two main forms of mental illness are recognisable; less severe forms of disorder in which the individual recognises that he/she needs help and a more severe form in which the affected person lacks insight into his/her health care needs and will not voluntarily seek such care. Moreover such individuals also lack mental capacity and may be at risk of abuse, neglect, rejection, discrimination and unfair practices by members of society. Conversely, those who suffer from severe mental illness may harm themselves, harm other people, or destroy property. When individuals lack capacity and insight into their mental state on account of severe mental illness treatment has to be given without the consent of the person under the provisions of the law. The purpose of the law, The Mental Treatment Act (MTA) is to ensure that individuals who suffer from severe mental illness receive care, protection and treatment while protecting people and property from potential harm resulting from mental illness. The MTA was first published on 31st August 1938 and was last revised in 1998. The MTA is outdated and criminalises mental illness and its management but continues to be used. This chapter outlines the relevant sections of the MTA, Chapter 279 of the Laws of Uganda.

Section 2

1. A magistrate inquires into the mental condition of a person suspected to be of unsound mind.
2. Inquiry is conducted as though the individual of unsound mind had committed an offence.
3. The magistrate may order that the individual suspected to be of unsound mind be brought before him/her for his/her personal inspection and examination.

4. Where the magistrate cannot inquire into the mind of the suspected mentally unsound person, he/she may order the detention of the said individual for safe custody, care and protection for a period of not more than 14 days.

5. The individual in respect of whom an order has been signed is detained for safe custody and care.

6. Inquiry is continued during the 14-day period before a magistrate in whose jurisdiction the individual of unsound mind may be detained.

7. The person suspected of being of unsound mind is released if found to be of sound mind.

8. Where an individual is dangerous to him/herself or others or is neglected and not cared for, the person who is responsible for the individual of unsound mind makes a report to a magistrate, chief or police officer so as to institute the process of inquiry into the mind of the person suspected to be of unsound mind.

Section 3

The magistrate appoints two medical practitioners not related to the suspected mentally disordered person and not in business partnership to independently examine and separately issue a report on the mental condition of the suspect.

Section 4

On the basis of the two medical reports the magistrate may issue a reception order authorizing the admission of the mentally disordered suspect to a gazetted mental hospital for the purpose of providing safety, custody, protection and care.

Section 5

Relatives of an individual suspected to be of unsound mind apply to the magistrate to have the person admitted to a mental hospital as a private paying patient.

Section 6

In the interest of public safety and the protection of the suspected mentally ill, any police officer not below the rank of Assistant Inspector of Police, a medical practitioner, or a chief, may cause the admission of the person under an urgency order for a period of 10 days for the purpose of observation before formal inquiry into his/her mental condition can be carried out.

Section 7

The magistrate signs a reception order to have the individual found to be of unsound mind conveyed to a mental hospital.

Section 8

A reception order lasts for a period of one year initially, then a further one year, followed by durations of three years at a time thereafter. The Medical Superintendent of the hospital is required to make reports to the Chief Registrar of the High Court for submission to the magistrate who signed the reception order on the mental and physical condition of the person concerned.

Section 9

The Chief Medical Officer is the sole officer authorized to be in charge of mental hospitals.

Section 10

Relatives of a suspected mentally disordered person admitted to hospital under section 8 are required to provide for the up-keep of the person in hospital.

Section 11

The funds for the up-keep of a mentally ill person in the mental hospital can be charged on his/her estate if such a person has sufficient funds available on the estate.

Section 13

Every person admitted to a mental hospital is under the control of the officers and servants of the hospital.

Section 14

Any person admitted to a mental hospital is required to remain in the hospital until he/she dies, or is discharged, or is transferred to another hospital or is sent home on leave.

Section 17-18

A person who has been admitted to a mental hospital may be discharged by the Chief Medical Officer upon the recommendation of the Medical Superintendent before the expiry of one year if the person has recovered from the mental disorder.

Section 19

A patient admitted on application of relatives may be discharged at their request.

Section 20

A patient may be sent home on leave from hospital at the discretion of the Medical Superintendent to ascertain the suitability for eventual discharge of the individual. If the person does not return to hospital within the specified period of leave the hospital is entitled to retake him/her without the issuance of a fresh reception order.

Any patient who escapes from the mental hospital without official discharge may be retaken to the hospital by an police officer, or staff of the hospital, or any other public servant within 28 days without the issuance of further reception order or certification on the authority of the Chief Medical Officer.

Sections 24-26

The Minister of Health appoints two or more official visitors in respect of every mental hospital. Visitors visit each hospital at least once every three months for the purpose of inspecting hospital records in respect of any patient to ascertain the welfare of patients, the reasons and justifications for hospitalisation of any patient and to make a report to the Minister of Health at the end of each visitation.

Sections 27-34

A variety of offences are stipulated to protect mentally ill persons and these include physical assault, sexual assault, ill treatment of patients, aiding the escape of mentally patients from hospital, selling articles to patients and trespassing on hospital grounds.

Section 41

The section provides for the protection of individuals who are involved in implementing the Act.

Section 42

Any mentally ill individual may raise complaints before the magistrate against anyone for any act done under the Act in the course of his/her detention in a mental hospital.

Section 46

Any mentally ill person may appeal to the High Court against his/her admission to a mental hospital within 30 days of such admission.

Comment

The MTA though recently revised remains outdated as are most of its provisions that govern the provision of care and treatment to people with mental disorder are adhered to. The Act treats the mentally sick as criminal aspects, does not protect the autonomy and rights of persons with mental disorder and does not allow for informal care and or aftercare following discharge from hospital. The MTA as it currently stands discriminates against persons with mental disorder and it does not provide for equal status between mental health and physical health care systems. Other laws exist that are relevant to mental health and these needs to be linked to any new MTA; including:

- The Penal Code Act provides for the assessment and treatment of persons who face prosecution for various offences in courts of law, but who show signs of mental ill-health.
- The Magistrates' Courts Act enables convicted prisoners who develop signs of mental ill-health in prison to receive psychiatric care in the course of their stay in prison.

- The 1995 Constitution provides for the assessment of the mental condition of any serving President or other senior ranking officers in government service to ascertain their mental fitness to remain in office.
- The Children's Statute provides for the welfare, care, and protection of children and adolescents but no specific clause that provides for their mental health exists.
- The Domestic Relations Bill does not provide for the mental health of partners in marriage and it is not clear how a partner whose mental health might be responsible for marital problems can access appropriate assessment and care for mental disorder.

It might be beneficial if any future MTA would provide for domiciliary care and recognise the role of several categories of health care providers (social worker, clinical psychologist, occupational therapist, mental health nurse, and psychiatric clinical officer) in providing care within the community on the basis of informal care when admission to hospital is not essential. Finally any new law should promote the equality of mental health care delivery system to the same status as the provision of care for physical conditions.

38
Mental Health Services and Referral Points

EMILIO OVUGA

The following are the Mental Health Services and skills available in the Health System by facility level in Uganda where mental health services can be accessed.

- Community / Health Centre I: There is a Community Health Worker (CHW) who is able to offer basic advice and support. The CHW can be trained to conduct follow-up services on behalf of the health center. If there are no such persons in the catchments, it may be advisable to train one.
- Health Centre II: There is a comprehensive Enrolled Nurse who has knowledge of mental health.
- Health Centre III: There is Comprehensive Registered Nurse with knowledge and skills in mental health.
- Health Centre IV: There is Medical Officer, Clinical Officers, and Comprehensive Registered and psychiatric nurses all of who can provide primary mental health service.
- District Hospital: There are Integrated mental health Services with some inpatient facility and psychiatric clinical officers as well as psychiatric nurses.
- Regional Hospital: There is an out patient and in patient services for Mental Health, headed by a Psychiatric Clinical Officer under supervision of a Psychiatrist
- National Referral Hospital: This offers tertiary referral, specialist psychiatric services.

Note: The referral system levels should be:

- The first referral point for any patient with mental disorders should be at health Centre IV. In some cases Health Center IV may also be the district hospital.
- The second referral point for any patient with mental disorders is the District Hospital.
- The third referral point for any patient with mental disorders is the Regional Hospital.
- The Tertiary referral is the National Referral Hospital at Butabika and Mulago Hospitals.

39
The Role of the Family in the Provision of Health Care

EMILIO OVUGA

Introduction

The family is the smallest unit in society and has traditionally comprised of two systems in Uganda; the nuclear family system comprises of husband, wife and their biological child or children, and the extended family system comprises of the nuclear system plus in-laws, aunts and uncles from the husband's and wife's side who may or may not live in the same neighbourhood for a variety of reasons. The extended family system is the most common though the influence of education, modernisation, rapid economic change and war and conflict are exerting powerful pressures to change this in favor of the nuclear family system. Table 1 below depicts some of the characteristics of the two family systems relevant for mental health. (See Table 1)

Some problems with mental illness

- Mental health problems tend to persevere or become chronic. This does not go down well with traditional concept of cure that is expected to result from only one episode of contact with health care system, whether native or otherwise.
- Severe forms of mental illness lead to loss of ability to recognise the need for one to seek or accept care and treatment. This problem leads to the worsening of the condition of those who suffer from severe mental illness. Thus it is then erroneously believed that mental illness is incurable and that once someone becomes mentally sick then he/she loses human values and is rejected forthwith by the family, relatives and community.
- Mental illness is surrounded by lack of information to the public regarding its treatment and prevention, and the ways for one to continue as well as regarding how to stay well following treatment.

Table 39.1: Characteristics of the nuclear and extended family systems in Uganda

Family system	Advantages	Disadvantages
Nuclear family system	• Income and other resources are usually adequate • Offspring theoretically receive the full attention of both parents • Permits the growth and development of personal autonomy within the context of the collective group	• Family members more likely to lack social support in the face of the pressures of daily living • In-laws and other relatives may be the source of conflict • Family members may lack emotional support offered by extended family system • Offspring may grow up not being informed of who their significant other relatives might be • Offspring may not be aware of their cultural heritage
Extended family system	• Emotional support and Counselling are readily available during crises • Social support is guaranteed • Material support is usually available at the time of need • Elders, aunts and uncles conduct informal cultural education for youth • Other family members freely substitute care for children • Emphasizes the community-rootedness of human nature • Burden of one member is the burden of everyone else	• In-laws sometimes fuel marital problems and compound family discord • Resources may not be adequate to meet the needs of all family members • Discourages individualism • Discourages personal initiative likely to lead to advancement beyond other members of one's group

- Because of its chronic nature mental illness tends to become expensive to treat. Poorly treated mental illness leads to emotional strain on family and relatives, loss of capacity for work, and financial strain, particularly if the breadwinner is the one who becomes mentally sick.

It is worthwhile to note that all these and other problems associated with mental illness can be controlled. The roles of the family in this regard are outlined below. First it should be recognised that the family is the only place in the life of its members that offers a safe environment. However the family may also be the most hazardous place to live in as a result of harmful patterns of relationships between its members. The provision of mental health care requires that families be helped by the health care provider to recognise their specific roles in the promotion of the wellbeing of its members and the prevention of new episodes of mental disorder.

The roles

- Family members are often the best placed to detect early signs of mental illness the first of which is change in behaviour.
- Family members can support the suspected mentally ill to accept the fact of illness.
- The family is often the one that seeks care and treatment for their mentally sick.
- The family should be helped to accept the mentally sick member and permit him/her to participate in the normal activities of the family. This helps the individual feel valued and motivated to prove their worth in life in spite of illness.
- The family can be taught the skills of supervision of medication at home along with monitoring changes in clinical behaviour.
- If the individual has no access to finances the family can provide transport money to support the individual's continued use of follow-up services.
- The family can be requested to participate in discussion of patterns of interpersonal relationships and other potential factors in mental illness.

40

The Role of the Community in the Delivery of Mental Health Services

John Wakida

Introduction

Community psychiatry refers to the body of knowledge and theories that are used to provide psychosocial services for individuals with mental disorders, neurological problems and behavioural disorders, outside the hospital environment in the community.

Aims

The aims of community psychiatry are to promote mental health, prevent mental illness, facilitate the access of communities to psychosocial services, and to prevent relapse among individuals who have recovered from active mental illness episodes. In the context of Uganda, community psychiatry aims to operationalize the integration of mental health services into general health care in the districts through the minimum health care package.

Components

Community psychiatry comprises a variety of activities whose ultimate aim is to provide services to individuals with psychosocial, neurological, and behavioural disorders, and these activities include:

- Acute short stay in-patient treatment at a facility within the individual's community setting, which does not last any longer than two to three days. The purpose of this service is to provide for the control of acute behavioural disturbance and for observation, thus obviating the need for formal hospitalisation with its possible subsequent stigmatization.
- Out-patient treatment services to provide for the evaluation of mental health problems for new comers, review of old patients, and provision of maintenance drug supplies.

- Residential Housing to provide alternative housing for the chronic mentally ill who might have been rejected by their families and usual social support systems, and have no housing of their own.
- Half-way housing facility for individuals who have been discharged from hospital, but may not be ready to return to their homes immediately, and who need further observation and treatment under health care staff supervision.
- Day care centers to provide psychosocial and medical care to individuals on outpatient basis. This service is for individuals who do not have sufficient social support to supervise medication at home. In addition the service provides opportunity for affected persons to interact with other individuals outside their own family.
- Rehabilitation and social re-integration services to help resettle individuals with long history of severe mental illness back into their communities.

A suggested model

It is expected that once mental health care has been fully integrated into the minimum health care package, psychosocial services will be provided from the district hospital level to the village level. The provision of such care will run through a cascade of care from the most rudimentary at village level through a system of referrals to the district hospital level.

The quality of services at the lower levels will be ensured through a system of support supervision of lower level health workers by higher level experienced health workers from the national referral hospital at Butabika Mental Hospital through the Regional Hospital down to the village level. It is expected that psychosocial services will be provided by health care workers together with welfare officers, clinical psychologists, occupational therapists, families and village health workers. It is recommended that appropriate village rehabilitation centers, and family support groups to foster the social and economic re-integration of former mentally ill persons into their communities will be established. It is expected that a functional community psychiatry program will work with traditional healers under the appropriate policy of the Ministry of Health to promote access to modern psychosocial services for persons who suffer from mental health problems, and to foster collaboration among modern mental health professionals and traditional healers.

Functions of community psychiatry program

The following are the major functions of a community psychiatry program.

- Early detection and treatment of common mental disorders at community level, e.g. first episode psychosis, temporary shelter for cases of domestic violence
- Observation and emergency care for the acutely disturbed, e.g. suicide attempt, intoxication with alcohol and drugs
- Provision of continuation medication to individuals recently discharged from hospital, e.g. individuals with chronic severe mental illness
- Follow up of individuals recently discharged from hospital, e.g. individuals with severe mental illness
- Rehabilitation and social re-integration of former mentally ill individuals into their homes, e.g. individuals who have been in hospital with severe mental illness for periods exceeding three months

Required input

The input necessary to ensure the success of a community level psychosocial program include:

- Motivated personnel
- Positive administrative and managerial attitude toward mental health and mental illness
- Adequate financial investment in the mental health of the community
- Provision of adequate supplies of effective medicines
- Functional referral system
- Regular training of health care staff
- Research and sufficient financing of mental health research
- Appropriate legislation and policy

41

Mental Health Promotion and Prevention of Mental Disorders

John Wakida

Introduction

The Uganda National Health Policy stresses the importance of improving the quality of life. The promotion of mental health, prevention and treatment of mental disorders is one of the ways of realising this goal.

Importance of prevention in Mental Health

The benefits of efforts to prevent mental disorders are:

- Reducing the level of social dependence due to mental disorders
- Reducing the cost of health care associated with mental disorders
- Reducing on the burden of disease (WHO estimates that 12.5% of the global burden of disease is due to mental health problems)
- Reducing on stigmatisation associated with mental disorders.
- Enhancing law and order in relation to mental health issues.
- Fostering the psychosocial well-being of individuals, families and community at large.

Preventive measures of mental disorders

Certain Mental disorders are preventable and some factors may set off or worsen the disorders:

1. **Hereditary :** Young individuals should be encouraged to explore each other's background to ascertain any familial disease before committing themselves into intimate relationships and marriage.

   Those already in relationships should be given Counselling and guidance on how best they can cope with the likely implications.

2. **Prevention of Infections**

   a) There should be immunisation against the six killer diseases.
   b) There should be improved sanitary conditions of the community.
   c) There should be early detection and proper treatment of those infections like Malaria, Meningitis, HIV etc, which are likely to cause mental disorders.

3. **There should be improved services Pregnancy and Birth**

   a) Encourage early and regular use of ante-natal services in order to prevent physical complications that would lead to mental health problems to the mother and the child. During the antenatal services psychological support should also be given to enable mothers to handle stress so that they do not develop mental disorders during the peuperium period.
   b) Encourage mothers to have supervised deliveries to avoid birth trauma to the newborn.

4. **Responsible Up-bringing of children**

   a) Reduces emotional deprivation, which may occur when infants and children are not given adequate loving care in institutions such as family, day-care centers, orphanages and hospitals.
   b) Helping children and adolescents develop healthy attitudes, by encouraging inquiry and discovery, self reliance, self confidence, and ability to cope with life situations independently especially at schools and homes.

5. **Healthy aging**

   a) To prepare the elderly cope with late life period. This may be achieved through reactivation, revival and protection of the cultural systems of social support that assures the elderly of care protection food shelter, etc.
   b) With the increasing modernisation of society it may be advisable for health care providers to advocate and lobby for policies and services for the elderly payable by the taxpayer.

6. **Encourage good nutrition**

   It is important to have proper and adequate nutrition in order to boost immunity and intellectual ability. Poor immunity will result

7. **Develop stress coping mechanism**

Stress can lead to mental disorders; individuals at workplace, and students should be empowered with life skills to be able to efficiently deal with the day-to-day challenges.

8. **Control of Substance Abuse (drugs and alcohol)**

Drugs of abuse when taken cause mental disorders, therefore there is need to: -

- Avoid substance of abuse.
- Enforce the law on illicit drug use.
- Do Counselling and guidance for potential substance abusers.
- Detect and treat any mental disorder that might be predisposing to the use of habit forming substances.

9. **Emergency and disaster preparedness**

Disasters of all forms cause severe and long lasting mental disorders with crippling symptoms such as anxiety, depression and proneness to suicide behaviour.

a) There is need to be prepared for natural and man-made disasters to avoid the resulting mental disorders.
b) Encourage mutual existence and respect for the opinions of other citizens regardless of the differences in politics, religion, tribe and social class.

10. **Prevention of Road Traffic Accident**

a) Protective helmets while riding motorcycle or while working at construction sites.
b) Use of seatbelts in motor vehicles
c) Taking measures to prevent domestic accidents involving both adults and children such as:
    - Accidental poisoning
    - Erection of physical barriers
    - Safeguarding fire-place in homes
d) Avoiding drunken driving
e) Teaching and enforcement of the Road Safety Act to the public and in schools.

11. Health Education Talk

Mental Health Education (MHE) is a basic foundation in prevention of Mental Disorders; therefore every health worker should endeavor to give MHE talks whenever he/she is in contact with clients and community.

Procedures to be followed

- Identify the target group.
- Choose a topic of discussion and explore more about it.
- Prepare how you are going to present it i.e. the resources you may require.
- Prepare your presentation in the following order:-
  - Introduction.
  - Objectives
  - Content
  - Summary.

1. Determine the methodology to use, depending on your target groups e.g. adult learning methods.
2. Communicate the information that you intend to convey to your audience, proposing the date, time and venue then confirm with them.
3. Conduct the education talk.
4. Evaluate.
5. Make a report for future modifications of the message and methods to use.

Remember that the main reason of preventing mental disorders is to promote the subjective sense of wellbeing amongst people and increase the participation of people in the full range of social and economic activities that give them a sense of purpose and meaning in life that may be associated with sense of good quality of life and increased productivity in the family, the community and the nation as a whole.

42
Psychiatric Emergencies

EMILIO OVUGA

A psychiatric emergency is a situation in mental health requiring immediate attention to avoid possible death, self-harm or harm to other people. Psychiatric emergencies require immediate attention as they cause a danger to the person, community and or property. It is therefore imperative that Health workers remain alert all the time to be able to protect the patient, communities and property from harm or destruction.

Disorders and situations causing psychiatric emergencies

Psychiatric emergencies usually occur in the context of mental disorders, which can be recognised whether at home or in hospital. The clinical condition of the patient is a key determinant as to whether a condition is an emergency or not. The following are mental disorders that may be associated with psychiatric emergency.

- Major depressive disorder
- Acute organic psychosis (delirium and delirium tremens may cause exhaustion, dehydration, harm)
- Postpartum psychosis (may lead to infanticide)
- Schizophrenia (paranoid schizophrenia; schizophrenic excitement)
- Manic excitement (exhaustion, dehydration)
- Personality disorder, e.g. anti-social personality disorder, paranoid personality disorder may lead to harm to others
- Drug intoxication may lead to harm
- Delinquency
- Post-ictal confusion in epilepsy
- Chronic organic brain syndrome
- Aggressive psychopaths
- Situational; psychiatric emergencies may be triggered by specific situations that may or may not be related to a person's mental disorder.

General Principles of Management of Psychiatric Emergencies

1. The patient should be attended to as soon as possible and relatives should be reassured.
2. Panic on the part of the staff worries the relatives more and may worsen the patients' symptoms, thus the need to be calm.
3. Initial treatment should focus on providing relief of acute and distressing symptoms. Treatment of the cause of the emergency can wait till later.
4. Some conditions have similar symptoms. It is important to differentiate between these conditions so that correct treatment may be given for the appropriate disorder.
5. Note that the psychiatric emergencies can reoccur, therefore, it is important that health education talks be given to the patient, relative, workmates/classmates and where possible follow-up for prevention of such recurrences.

A Health worker should look out for following conditions:-

1. Attempted suicide
2. Aggressive and violent behaviour (Acute psychotic states)
3. Status epilepticus (this is not a mental disorder but a neurological condition, which is best managed by a physician)
4. Rape and defilement
5. Child disappearing from home

Suicide behaviour

Suicide behaviour is a spectrum of human behaviour that may lead to a person killing him or herself, and comprises of the following elements

- Wish to die
- Wish to commit suicide
- Communication of the intention to commit suicide
- Making suicide plan
- Execution of suicide plan

- Suicide attempt
- Completed suicide

Prevalence

80 people commit suicide every hour worldwide. Up to 40% of the general population experience the wish to die at least once in their lifetime. The World Health Organisation estimates that by the year 2020, there will be one suicide every 20 seconds and one suicide attempt every 1-2 seconds (Bertolote, 2001).

Suicide is common in Uganda though the rate may vary from region to region, and from sub-county to sub-county. In one sub-county in Adjumani district the rate of suicide has been estimated at 99 per 100,000 inhabitants in 2003, and the rate of suicide attempt was estimated to be 518 per 100,000 inhabitants in 2002. In 2004 the estimated rate for suicide in the whole district of Adjumani was 49.6 per 100,000 inhabitants and that of attempted suicide, 50.1 per 100,000 inhabitants. At least 15% of the population in Uganda have a previous history of suicide attempt (Ovuga, 2005) and 16% of the adult population report the experience of suicide behaviour in the past year (Kanarukara et al, 2004).

Aetiology

- 90% of suicides occur within the context of a mental disorder, particularly depression; suicide behaviour can occur in the context of any mental disorder.
- Difficulties in interpersonal relationships.
- Adverse socio-economic circumstances.
- Chronic physical illness, e.g. cancer, HIV/AIDS, congestive cardiac failure.

Attempted suicide

Suicide attempt may occur in the following conditions and situation:

1. Depressive illness
2. Schizophrenia
3. Panic (anxiety) disorder
4. Chronic organic brain syndrome
5. Under the influence of alcohol and/or drugs

6. Manic disorder
7. Post-traumatic stress disorder
8. Following rape/defilement

Common methods used for committing suicide

- Ingesting poison
- Jumping from a height, hanging and inhaling poisonous gases.
- Drowning
- Self starvation.

High risk Factors

- Negative ideas about life – hopelessness, lack of meaning in life
- Feeling of social rejection, abandonment, lack of social support system
- Presence of mental illness, particularly depression
- Presence of suicide behaviour
- Previous history of suicide attempt
- Family history of suicide attempt or completed suicide
- Presence of general medical illness

Other Risk Factors

- Sex – more males commit suicide than females
- Age – those aged more than 44 years tend to commit rather than attempt suicide.
- Alcohol – concomitant alcohol or other drug abuse raise the risk of suicide.
- Loss of rational thinking – the loss of rational thinking, as occurs in delirium, schizophrenia or manic excitement raises the risk of suicide.
- The presence of interpersonal difficulties including marital difficulties in Uganda is associated with high risk of successful suicide.
- Evidence of organised plan is associated with high risk of successful suicide.
- Recent loss of status, role, and esteem in social relationships predisposes to successful suicide.
- Poverty and unemployment – suicide is a disease of poverty.
- Circumstances of a previous or planned suicide bid – if the individual attempted, or plans to carry out a suicide act when rescue was/is unlikely, then the risk of successful suicide is very high.

- Timing - most successful suicides occur after midnight or mid-morning when rescue from a suicide bid is unlikely.
- Method - the choice of a hard method such as hanging points to a high risk of successful suicide.
- Communication of suicide wish - Communication of suicide intent is one of the most powerful predictors of successful suicide. Remember, though, that communication of suicide intent may be intended to elicit last minute help from close social contacts; the motive of communication should therefore be evaluated adequately. The communication of suicide intent may be direct or subtle.
  - Direct communication: "If you think that I am not the head of this home, I will leave this world for you."
  - Indirect communication: "I am fed up with life." I wish I were not born."
- Suicide note - the presence of a suicide note for a previous attempt, or plan to leave a suicide note before executing a planned suicide act is associated with a high suicide risk.
- The absence of dependents or lack of specific responsibility for the welfare of other family members carries a high risk of suicide.
- Evaluation of failed suicide act - an individual who is disappointed with the failure of a suicide bid may attempt suicide again.

Assessing suicide risk

A highly suicidal patient:

- Is severely depressed or has overt signs of florid psychosis.
- Has attempted or tried to attempt suicide before coming to you.
- Has an urgent wish to die, possibly within a week or so; natural death is too far.
- Has an active plan for implementing suicide plan.
- Will feel disappointed if suicide bid fails.
- May have communicated the suicide intention to some one else.

Remember that suicide risk remains substantial up to three months after apparent clinical recovery. Suicide prevention measures should therefore remain in force and the patient should be monitored regularly for suicide potential. The best precaution to take in suicide prevention and suicide risk assessment is to detect suicide potential proactively in every high risk

Management of suicide behaviour

- Detect suicide behaviour in every patient with clinical interview. Up to 46% of the general population have suicide ideation (Ovuga et al, 2005).
- Determine the risk of suicide occurring.
- Detect the presence of a psychiatric disorder, particularly depression, or chronic general medical illness or psycho-social stressors.
- Develop treatment and suicide prevention plan with patient and carer.
- Educate the patient and carer about suicide behaviour.
- Suicide behaviour is a normal human experience.
- Suicide behaviour can be treated.
- Talking about death, dying and suicide helps people to drop the suicide idea.
- Start medication for appropriate psychiatric disorder.
- Discuss the prevention of suicide behaviour with colleague in-charge of general medical care (as appropriate).
- Enter into a contract with the patient so that he/she can contact carer, friend, or yourself in case he/she experiences the suicide urge.
- Start cognitive therapy aimed at reducing the patient's irrational and negative ideas, beliefs, and attitudes and, at teaching the patient effective problem-solving skills as described in item 10 below.
- Help the patient solve or cope with interpersonal problems or current and ongoing psychosocial stressor. Gently guide the patient to :
- Narrate the nature of his/her current and ongoing life difficulties.
- Describe his/her previous, current and ongoing psycho-social stressors.
- Evaluate the meaning and significance of his/her difficulties and psychosocial stressors In relation to his/her aspirations, plans and hopes in life.
- Develop a hierarchy of his/her usual responses to life stressors.
- Evaluate the effectiveness of each of these responses.
- Develop alternative responses and strategies to solve his/her difficulties.
- Develop homework for the patient to carry out.
- Evaluate the outcome of the implementation of home work assignments and identify problems and obstacles the patient encountered; discuss how the patient could get round the identified problems, etc.

- Dispense drugs on weekly basis only till the risk of suicide has substantially been removed.
- If in doubt refer to the psychiatrist, psychologist or professional counsellor early.

Prevention of suicide behaviour

The prevention of suicide should be the task of every health worker. The prevalence of suicide behaviour can be reduced through:

- Early detection of suicide ideas among patients.
- Early detection of depression.
- Effective treatment of disorders associated with suicide.
- Improve prescription habits that promote safety in psychotropic drug use.
- Improving general socio-economic situation of communities.

Caution in case of suicide behaviour

- Every suicide attempt should be taken seriously as a successful attempt may follow thereafter.
- The patient is often unmanageable in an out-patient setting, therefore, requires hospitalisation.
- The patient should be under close observation; potentially harmful materials such as drugs, sharp objects should be removed.
- If suspected to have taken poison, close observation and antidote for poison should be given.
- When the patients life is no longer in immediate danger from suicide, a health worker should talk to the patient to understand the reasons why the patient was attempting suicide.
- A health worker should adopt an understanding rather than a punitive or judgmental working attitude.
- The underlying psychotic disorders e.g. depression or schizophrenia should be managed appropriately.

Aggressive and violent behaviour

Psychiatric emergency may take the form of aggressive behaviour, which may be unprovoked and is usually directed at family members. In this case the aggression may be in response to delusions that the victim is behind the sick person's continued illness or in protest against being taken to traditional healers or being locked up in a room alone. Frequently aggression may be provoked by members of the general public through insults directed at the mentally ill who may be passing by.

- Schizophrenia
- Acute organic syndrome especially alcohol intoxication, drug intoxication and delirium.

Management of aggressive behaviour

- In the case of the hospitalised patient do not take him/her by surprise, explain all the procedures you are going to do; assure the individual of his/her security
- It is important for a health worker not to become frightened or excited as this may reduce the effectiveness of any measures taken and interfere with finding a rational solution to a problem.
- There should be quick organised intervention to avoid injury to self and others, however, if you are alone seek help from others.
- A health worker should try to understand why a patient is aggressive before resorting to restraining methods.
- Enough human resources should be readily available.
- Be aware of the patient with aggression and show them that you are in control of the situation.
- In case of an armed patient, he should be disarmed without causing harm. During the process, do not all talk at once, let the person with the best relationship with the aggressive/violent individual do the talking in a calm and convincing manner.
- Never approach an aggressive mental patient alone.
- Use minimal restraint when necessary and discontinue when it is no longer necessary.
- Once the incident is over, follow up the patient to establish the possible cause of the behaviour.

- Incase of organic brain syndrome, identify the physical cause and manage it accordingly. This type of patients require extra care for which you should refer to (Unit 6.1 organic mental disorder) for detailed appropriate management.

Status Epilepticus

These are repeated attacks of generalised, tonic, clonic seizures without gaining consciousness in between. These may be caused by

- Sudden withdrawal of anti-epileptic drugs
- Infections
- Sudden stressful situations
- Starvation
- Excessive exhaustion
- Hormonal changes.

Management of status epilepticus

- Remove the patient from danger
- Loosen tight clothing
- Do not restrain the jerking
- Clear airway
- Do not give anything by mouth
- Place the patient in lateral position
- Refer to hospital for further management including investigations within 12 hours.

Caution in case of status epilepticus

Do not place anything between teeth during the attack, as this may injure the patients' gums.

Drugs in status epilepticus

- Diazepam 10 mg rectally (See details in the chapter on epilepsy)

Rape and defilement

Rape is defined as having sexual (carnal) knowledge of a woman without her consent. Defilement refers to having sexual relations with a female person under the age of 18 years. Though rape and defilement may also involve males and boys as victims of both adult women and men much of the attention remains focused on women and girls as victims of men; note also that adult women as perpetrators of the rape and defilement of women and girls has hardly been reported in the local press in Uganda. Apart from the physical injuries inflicted on the survivor, there are associated emotional and psychosocial effects of the trauma. However whereas the physical injuries are given due attention the emotional and psychosocial sequelae are not taken care of though these often lead to short and long-term mental health effects on victims.

Physical effects of rape and defilement

- Injuries/bruises of the private and/other parts.
- Bleeding excessively
- Infection, HIV/Syphilis/gonorrhea
- Unwanted pregnancy

Psychological effects of rape and defilement

- Fear and anxiety
- Depression
- Stigma
- Self guilt/blame
- Sleeplessness due to nightmares
- Re-experiencing the event rape
- Numbing of emotions
- Worthlessness, hopelessness and helplessness
- Feeling dirty
- May develop obsessive compulsive behaviour
- They may develop fear of the men in the case of women victims

Management of rape and defilement

It should be a comprehensive package, which involves:

- Counseling by experienced Counsellor
- Respect for confidentiality
- Treating physical complications such as injuries and infections
- Follow up and home visiting
- In case of pregnancy refer to appropriate Counsellor
- Ensure protection of the survivor from future abuse through life-skills training.

43
Psychological Methods of Therapy

EMILIO OVUGA

Introduction

Psychological methods of treating mental health problems involve conversations also known as "talk therapy". The table 1 below depicts a classification of talk therapies that may be employed in treating people with mental or general health problems in primary health care, particularly alcohol abuse problems, suicide behaviour, depression, anxiety and the psychological complications of domestic violence, rape, armed conflict and war. Counselling, the less sophisticated form of talk therapy, may be used in the routine care of individuals with a variety of physical conditions ranging from life-threatening disorders such as cancer, HIV/AIDS to acute infections such as malaria and lobar pneumonia.

Table 43.1: Classification of psychological methods of therapy

Quality	Counselling	Psychotherapy
Classification	• Supportive Counselling • Dynamic Counselling	• Supportive psychotherapy • Psychoanalysis • Cognitive psychotherapy • Behavioural psychotherapy • Interpersonal psychotherapy

Application	• General medical conditions, e.g. cancer, HIV/AIDS, tuberculosis, diabetes mellitus, hypertension • Crisis situations, e.g. domestic violence, conflict and war, rape, suicide behaviour • Mental disorders, e.g. depression, anxiety disorders, alcohol dependence • Chronic mental disorder, e.g. schizophrenia, manic disorder	• General medical conditions, e.g. cancer, HIV/AIDS, tuberculosis, diabetes mellitus, hypertension • Crisis situations, e.g. domestic violence, conflict and war, rape, suicide behaviour • Mental disorders, e.g. depression, anxiety disorders • Chronic mental disorder, e.g. schizophrenia, manic disorder • Personality disorders
Users	• All health care providers • Counsellors	• Psychiatrists • Psychotherapists • Professional Counsellors

Counselling

Counselling is a form of conversations that helps a person affected by psychological, social, economic, or other problem of living to examine their feelings, thinking behaviour, interpersonal relationships and purpose in life. Counselling creates self-awareness, helps the individual understand the reasons for his/her problems, leads to a development of healthy ways of dealing with personal problems and personal growth, and enables the individual to face future problems successfully. Counselling may be conducted at individual level (Individual Counselling) or for groups of persons at the same time (Group Counselling) or for couples who are experiencing marital difficulties (Couple and family therapy). Several techniques are used in the course of Counselling and these include listening, reassurance, education, guidance, instruction, advice, and material assistance where as indicated, e.g. the provision of crutches wheelchair or prosthesis.

Counselling in a rural traditional environment depends on the type of problem that the individual is experiencing and it occurs within the overall provision of traditional health care. Broadly problems in this type of care are categorized into three; those that:

a) Occur as a result of natural negative events and are not within an individual's control, e.g. depression or anxiety disorder following bereavement, infertility, unemployment

b) Are the outcome of an individual's actions or omissions, e.g. possession state following involvement in acts of atrocities, the murder of someone

c) Were sent by a person's enemies, e.g. psychosis

The types of Counselling offered under each of these categories are depicted in the table 2 that follows.

Table 43.2: Types of Counselling services offered in traditional medicine

Natural negative life events	**Outcome of personal actions, omissions**	**The result of actions by one's enemies**
Provide emotional support, encourage expression of grief over loss, e.g. mourning rituals	Fulfill personal obligations and responsibilities to the family and clan spirits	Cast out evil spirits
Give company; do not leave alone e.g. visits from friends who encourage self-disclosure and provide company	Performance of customary rituals	Sacrifice animal prescribe by the evil spirits
Reassure, e.g. that you are not alone, everything will be alright, it was not your fault	Offer sacrifice to ancestral spirits	Plant medicinal products to keep evil spirits away
Engage in group activities, e.g. social gathering, gardening	General behaviour conforming to prescription made by healer	Wearing of medicinal products to protect health against the evil
Give material assistance, e.g. food, clothing, money	Participation in drama (to encourage release of emotional tension)	Participation in drama (to encourage release of emotional tension)

Psychotherapy

Psychotherapy is a specialised form of talk therapy that works the same way that Counselling does. Psychotherapy requires professional training for four years with supervision provided by senior psychotherapists before allowing the trainee practice on their own. There are several forms of psychotherapy each of which is founded on a specific theory; the firs form of psychotherapy founded by Sigmund Freud is known as classical psychoanalysis. The practice of psychoanalysis is based on the theory that every individual has in their unconscious part of the mind hidden childhood painful memories that continue to govern behaviour in the present. It is believed that symptoms of mental illness are the manifestations of these unpleasant painful memories, and that cure can be achieved only when these memories are brought to conscious awareness through the analysis of the symptoms of illness, dreams and behaviour in daily life and relating these to what one is able to recall from childhood.

Cognitive psychotherapy is based on the theory that people become depressed, or develop anxiety disorder because they view their world the wrong way round; that is, depressed individuals blame themselves because they undermine their potentials, underrate their achievements and magnify their faults. Cognitive therapy helps the individual with depression to examine them to discover the positive things in themselves leading to recovery from depressive illness.

Behaviour therapy assumes that symptoms of illness, like all behaviours are learned and that cure rests in unlearning symptoms of ill-health. Behaviour therapy is best used in the treatment of anxiety disorders

Interpersonal Therapy (IPT)

Introduction

Problems in relating with members of one's social network give rise to depression, suspicion, anxiety, alcohol abuse, suicide, etc. Cure for mental health problems require acquiring the necessary skills to correct faulty interpersonal relationships. Research in Uganda (Bolton and associates, 2004) and clinical field experience (Ovuga, unpublished) suggest that it is feasible to train lay persons to conduct interpersonal therapy for groups in primary care. This section describes the process of how this can be done.

Areas in interpersonal relationships

Interpersonal therapy (IPT) assumes that symptoms of mental disorder result from faulty interpersonal relationships characterised by unmet social and emotional needs, disputes, shyness, inability to negotiate solutions for personal difficulties and problems in moving from one social role and status to the next. There are four main areas in interpersonal relations, namely:

- Loss, grief; social isolation, loneliness
- Disputes; disagreements: problems in authority, status, role, responsibility
- Economic loss, poverty
- Life changes

One or more of these problem areas generate unpleasant thoughts and emotions that lead to unpleasant interpretations and expectations, which lead to faulty interpersonal relationships and aggravate negative emotions, other feelings and negative reactions with associated physical symptoms; these intensify the individual's original personal problem areas resulting in a vicious cycle. See figure 1 below that depicts what happens when a problem in interpersonal relationships arises.

Fig 43.1: Chain of events in interpersonal relationships

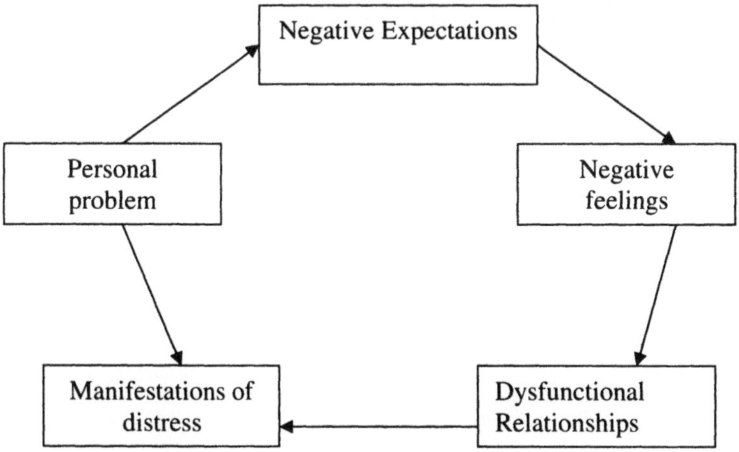

The process of Interpersonal Therapy

IPT may be conducted either for individuals or for groups through the following steps.

- Identify the main symptoms that the individual suffers from.
- Identify the nature of situations that precipitate distress symptoms.
- Identify and focus on aspects of situations that are under the direct control of the distressed individual.
- Draw linkages between feelings, experiences and any of the problem areas responsible for the person's distress symptoms.
- Draw a list of possible options that the individual can use to solve the presenting difficulty.
- Figure out which options might solve the stressful situation best.
- Build skills based on the selected options to solve the difficulty.
- Support the individual members with their own problems and the problems of other group members if you are running group IPT sessions.
- Identify potential sources of help including financial support, help from friends and relatives, etc.

Example

Study the following example of a man with alcohol use disorder and who survived a suicide attempt by over-dose. Generate your own solutions to this problem based on the IPT analysis. See table 3 that follows.

"My wife looks at me as a simple man because I am not working now and therefore I have no money now. She despises me, abuses me and does not listen to me or do what I tell her to do. I have anger due to my lack of money these days, and my wife's love seems to be fading. As a result she can love another man and leave me, or sleep with another man and bring us AIDS."

Table 43.3: Problem analysis in IPT

Problem area	Description
Personal problem	Loss of job; poverty Loss of role status Loss of authority status, respect
Expectations	Loss of love Fear of rejection Fear of HIV/AIDS
Dysfunctional relationships	Wife despises husband Poor sexual relations Ineffectual communication Verbal abuse
Emotions, feelings, reactions	Anger Sense of failure; life meaningless
Manifestations of distress	Alcohol abuse Suicide attempt
Possible solutions	• Clarify the man's problems • Clarify the man's expectations • Redefine the nature of marital sexual relationships • What other symptoms does the man experience • Clarify the problems from the wife's view point • Who could be engaged in therapy sessions?

Uses of IPT

IPT is basically problem-oriented and may be used in the following situations to help individuals get over the distressing problems of depression, anxiety, and suicide behaviour or alcohol abuse.

- IPT group replaces the family or social network when these are not working well for individual members
- IPT replaces lost social support systems

- IPT provides trusting atmosphere for distressed persons to share their personal problems
- IPT offers a process of enhancing problem-solving options for persons in difficulty.
- IPT may be used to engage families in resolving disputes and relationship problems.

Natural reactions to expect from the client

The following reactions that are common during the process of any talk therapy sessions may arise, and when they do, tact time and patience with appropriate support to the individual are required. Do not rush; absorb the reactions of the client without anger, feeling of failure shame or guilt on your part; avoid forcing the person into admitting distress if he/she is not yet ready (this will come when you list expect it); remain optimistic; let the client decide the pace of how much to say.

- Denial
- Disbelief, shock
- Anger, irritability
- Shame, blame, guilt
- Shyness
- Bargaining
- Issues of acceptance, dependence needs

Confidentiality

Community members often experience common problems and they tend to share personal troubles in the process of providing and securing social emotional support. It is likely that health care providers might have gone through the same experiences. Discovery of this situation should serve as reminder of the commonness of the human condition and as a source of strength for the health care provider. The health care provider should not however reveal information about the individual with emotional problems. In preparing to conduct talk therapy sessions with individuals:

- Ask if the individual would like conversations with you in the presence of other people including family

- Otherwise conduct conversations in private
- Assure the individual that you will not reveal information that you have acquired to other individuals
- In the case of potential suicide, inform the person that you will notify family about the danger of a possible suicide
- Explain the benefits of notifying or involving family in conversations regarding his/her health care

References

Arcel, L.T. (1998) War violence, trauma and the coping process: Armed conflict in Europe and survivor response, IRCT Publications, Copenhagen, Denmark

African Psycare Research Organisation (APRO) (1999) The psychological consequences of war traumatisation on the women of Luwero district, An Intervention Report to Isis-WICCE, Kampala, Uganda

Amundson, Kristen. (1993) *Speaking and Writing Skills for Educators*, Arlington, Virginia: American Association of School Administrators, Pg 20

Allwood C.W. & Gagiano CA (1997) *Handbook of Psychiatry for Primary Care*, Oxford, Oxford University Press.

APA (1992) *Diagnostic and Statistical Manual of Mental Disorders*, Washington DC, American Psychiatric Association

Bertolote JM (2001). Suicide in the world: an epidemiological overview, 1959-2000. In: Wasserman D (Ed). In: *Suicide: An Unnecessary Death*. Martin Dunitz, p6. Current opinion in psychiatry, Vol. 11(1), 1998

Boardman J. & Ovuga E. (1997) Rebuilding psychiatry in Uganda, *Psychiatric Bulletin*, **21:** 649-655.

Ovuga E. (1997). Overview of HIV/AIDS and mental health in Uganda, Parapraxis, **3(2):** 35-39.

Burton, T., & Mutiti, A (1998) *Northern Uganda Psychosocial Needs Assessment*, UNICEF, Marianum Press

Cookson J, Taylor D and Katona C (2002) Use Of Drugs In Psychiatry, Gaskell, 5th Edition, Cromwell Press Limited, U.K.

Covey, Stephen R. (1990) *The Seven Habits of Highly Effective People*. New York: Fireside Books, Simon and Schuster.

Daniel, Y. (1998) *International Handbook Of Multigenerational Legacies Of Trauma*, Plenum Press, New York

Gilbert, T., Performance engineering, In: *What Woks At Work: Lessons From The Masters*, Lakewood Books, Minneapolis, 1988, p.20.

Herman, J. (1997) Trauma and Recovery - from domestic abuse to political terror, Basic Books, New York

Isis-WICCE (August 2002) Medical interventional study of war affected women in Teso region, Uganda, Kampala

Jegede R.O.(1988) *Psychiatry For Health Professional;* Macmillan Publishers Ltd, London

Kendell R.E and Zealley A.K. (1988), *Companion to Psychiatric Studies* Churchhill Livingstone, Edinburgh.

Kinyanda, E. & Musisi, S (2001) War traumatisation and its psychological consequences in women of Gulu district, In: *Violnce Against Women And Children, Review Of Women's Studies,* Vol XI Nos. 1 and 2, University of Philippines

Kinyanda, E. & Musisi, S. (2000) *Psychiatric Problems of HIV/AIDS and their Management in Uganda,* Kampala - Manual

Margolis, F.H, and Bell, C.R. (1989) *Understanding Training: Perspectives and Practices,* University Associates, San Diego, pp 13-15.

Musisi, S., Kinyanda, E., Liebling, H., et al(2000) Post-traumatic torture disorders in Uganda: a three year retrospective study of patient records at a specialised torture treatment center in Uganda, Torture, 10(3):81-87

Maxmen JS and Ward NG (1995). Psychotropic Drugs - Fast Facts, Second edition W.W. Norton & Company, New York

Ngana Suvian (a) (1988) *Mental Health and Mental Illness,* John Wiley & Sons, New York

Odendi, G.R. (2005) *The Prevalence Of Alcohol Dependence Among Adults Admitted To Adjumani District Hospital,* Dissertation for the Diploma in Mental Health, School of Psychiatric Clinical Officers, Ministry of Education & Sports, Kampala

Ovuga, E. (2005) *Depression and Suicidal Behaviour in Uganda: Validating the Response Inventory for Stressful Life Events (RISLE),* PhD thesis, Karolinska Institute and Makerere University, Stockholm and Kampala

Ovuga, E. & Madrama, C (2006) The magnitude of alcohol use problems in the Uganda Police Force in Kampala District, *African Health Sciences,* March 2006

Ovuga, E., Boardman, J., & Wasserman, D (2005) Prevalence of depression in two districts of Uganda, *Social Psychiatry Psychiatric Epidemiology*, 40(6): 439-445

Ovuga, E., Boardman, J., & Wasserman, D (2005) Prevalence of suicide ideation in two districts of Uganda, *Archives of Suicide Research*,)9(4): 321-332

Orley, J. & Wing, J. (1979) Psychiatric disorders in two African villages, *Archives of General Psychiatry*, 36: 513-520

Petrushkin H, Boardman J & Ovuga E (2005 Psychiatric conditions in HIV positive individuals attending an AIDS Support Organisation (TASO) clinic in urban Kampala. *Psychiatric Bulletin*, 29: 451-458

Royal College of Psychiatrists (2000) *Good Psychiatric Practice 2000*, Royal College of Psychiatrists

Tomb D (ed) Post-traumatic stress disorder, In: *The Psychiatric Clinics Of North America*, Vol 4, Number 4, June 1994

United Nations (1991) *The Protection of Persons with Mental Illness and the Improvement of Mental Health Care* United Nations General Assembly, 75th plenary meeting, 17 December 1991

Walugembe, J. (1994) *Post-Traumatic Disorder Among Patients Attending Mulago Hospital*, Dissertation for Master of Medicine in Psychiatry, Department of Psychiatry, Makerere University, Kampala

WHO, Division of Mental Health, Geneva (1995) *Initiative of Support to People with Epilepsy*, Cambridge International Dictionary of English Cambridge University Press, London

WHO (1992) *International Classification of Diseases*, World Health Organisation, Geneva

Index

www.ingramcontent.com/pod-product-compliance
Ingram Content Group UK Ltd.
Pitfield, Milton Keynes, MK11 3LW, UK
UKHW040228290926
15471UKWH00001B/57

9 789970 026111